100 Data Interpretation Questions for the MRCP

100 Data Interpretation Questions for the MRCP

by
Richard Ashford
MA, MB, B.Chir., MRCP(UK)
Senior Medical Registrar,
St Stephen's Hospital,
London

and

Patrick Venables
MA, MB, B.Chir., MRCP(UK)
Research Fellow,
Charing Cross Hospital,
London

CHURCHILL LIVINGSTONE
EDINBURGH LONDON AND NEW YORK 1979

CHURCHILL LIVINGSTONE
Medical Division of Longman Group Limited

Distributed in the United States of America by
Longman Inc., 19 West 44th Street, New York,
N.Y. 10036, and by associated companies,
branches and representatives throughout
the world.

First Edition 1979

ISBN 0 443 01810 3

British Library Cataloguing in Publication Data

100 data interpretation questions for the MRCP.
    1. Diagnosis – Problems, exercises, etc.
    I. Ashford, Richard II. Venables, Patrick
    III. Hundred data interpretation questions for the
    MRCP
    616.07'5'076   RC71.3   78-40711

Printed in Singapore by
Kua Co., Book-Manufacturers Pte Ltd

Introduction

The aim of this book is to enable the reader to assess his or her ability to make deductions from laboratory data. We would not claim that data interpretation should be the sole means of assessing patients, but we do feel that, as the laboratory is acquiring increasing importance in diagnosis and management, a book devoted to investigations and their interpretation is justified.

The layout of the book is similar to that of the written section of the MRCP. The hundred questions are divided into ten 'papers' each consisting of 2 ECG's and eight other questions which include chemical pathology, haematology, lung function tests, blood gases and cardiac catheter data. Most of the questions and all of the ECG's are based on patients seen by us or our colleagues, though obviously some of the information has had to be altered slightly to enable fair questions to be asked. As a result some of the examples may seem rather artificial or perhaps too 'typical' to be real. Nevertheless, we feel that such an adjustment is necessary to ensure that none of the information is irrelevant or misleading.

In each case answers are provided and where relevant the differential diagnosis briefly discussed. The book is not intended to be a textbook and we hope that any information that is provided in the answers is used more as an aid in the technique of interpretation than as a source of factual knowledge. The veracity of every answer has been checked carefully and in this context we are particularly grateful to our colleagues for their helpful criticisms. In particular we would like to mention Dr J Silva who has reviewed the chemical pathology; Dr D Samson, the haematology and Dr R Sutton, the ECG's and catheter data. Others who have given either data or advice include Dr K Venables, Dr M Brenner, Dr P Butler and Dr A Scott-Keat. Our thanks go to Karen King, Angela Millen and Mary Wheeler for typing the manuscript.

We should also draw attention to the MRCP candidates who attended the course at St. Stephen's Hospital, London, where the contents of this book have been used as teaching material for the last 18 months. Their comments (not always lacking in emotion!) during our many sessions have helped enormously in the evolution of what we believe to be a fair and moderately testing collection of questions.

Table of normal ranges

Plasma or serum	SI Units	Conventional Units
Alanine transaminase ALT (SGPT)	0.20 U/l	0-20 U/l
Albumin	35-45 g/l	3.5-4.5 g/100 ml
Aldosterone	100-330 mmol/l	2.5-12 ng/100 ml
Alkaline phosphatase	20-100 U/l	3-12 King-Armstrong U/100 ml
Anti-Diuretic Hormone (ADH)		4-8 ng/l
Aspartate transaminase AST (SGOT)	0-25 U/l	0-25 U/l
Bicarbonate	22-28 mmol/l	22-28 mEq/l
Bilirubin	2-17 μmol/l	0.1-1 mg/100 ml
Calcium	2.25-2.62 mmol/l	9-10.6 mg/100 ml
Chloride	93-108 mmol/l	93-108 mEq/l
Cholesterol	3.6-7.2 mmol/l	145-280 mg/100 ml
Cortisol: 9 am	170-720 nmol/l	6-26 μg/100 ml
midnight	170-220 nmol/l	6-8 μg/100 ml
Creatinine phosphokinase (CPK)	$<$100 U/l	
Creatinine	$<$80 μmol/l	1.0mg/100 ml
DNA Binding	$<$25 U	
Growth hormone		$<$10 ng/ml
Glucose (fasting)	3.6-6.6 mmol/l	65-120 mg/100 ml
Immunoglobulins IgA	1.25-4.25 g/l	125-425 mg/100 ml
IgG	5-16 g/l	500-1600 mg/100 ml
IgM	0.5-1.7 g/l	50-170 mg/100 ml

I-131 uptake	11-33% of dose at 4 hours	
Iron:		
males	16-30 μmol/l	90-170 g/100 ml
females	11-27 μmol/l	60-150 g/100 ml
Iron binding capacity (TIBC)	45-72 μmol/l	250-400 g/100 ml
Magnesium	0.65-1 mmol/l	1.3-2.0 mEq/l
Osmolality (plasma)	285-295 mmol/l	285-295 (mosmols/l)
pCO_2	4.7-6.0 kPa	35-45 mmHg
pO_2	12-13.3 kPa	90-100 mmHg
pH		7.36-7.45
Phosphate	0.8-1.4 mmol/l	2.5-4.3 mg/100 ml
Potassium	3.5-5.0 mmol/l	3.5-5.0 mEq/l
Protein (total)	58-72 g/l	5.8-7.2 g/100 ml
Protein (CSF)	0.15-0.4 g/l	15-50 mg/100 ml
Serum hydroxy-butyric-dehydrogenase (SHBD)	50-170 U/l	
Sodium	133-145 mmol/l	133-145 mEq/l
Thyroxine (T4)	70-160 nmol/l	5.5-12.5 μg/100 ml
T3 Resin uptake	88-110%	
Thyroid stimulating hormone (TSH)	0.8-3.6 mU/l	
Urea	3.3-7.0 mmol/l	20-42 mg/100 ml
Urate:		
male	0.24-0.44 mmol/l	4.0-7.5 mg/100 ml
female	0.21-0.37 mmol/l	3.5-6.2 mg/100 ml
Faecal fat	0-17 mmol/24 hr	0-59/24 hr
Urine		
Coproporphyrins		<0.1 mg/24 hr
Hydroxy-methoxy-malonic acid	5-35 μmol/24 hr	1.7 mg/24 hr

Haematological

Haemoglobin (Hb):
males	13.5-18.0 g/dl	13.5-18.0 g/100 ml
females	11.5-16.5 g/dl	11.5-16.5 g/100 ml

Red blood cell count:
males	4500-6.500 x 10^9/l	4.5-6.5million/mm^3
females	3900-5600 x 10^9/l	3.9-5.6million/mm^3

Packed cell volume (PCV):
males	0.4-0.54	40-54 per cent
females	0.35-0.47	35-47 per cent

Mean corpuscular haemoglobin (MCH)	27-32 pg	27-32 ρg
Mean corpuscular haemoglobin concentration (MCHC)	32-36 g/dl	32-36 per cent
Mean corpuscular volume (MCV)	76-98 fl	76-98 νm^3
Reticulocyte count		0.2-2 per cent

White blood count (WBC)
	$\times 10^9$/l	/mm^3
total	4.0-11.0	4000-11000
neutrophils	2.5-7.5	2500-7500
lymphocytes	1.5-3.5	1500-3500
cosinophile	0.04-0.44	40-440
basophile	0-0.1	0-100
monocytes	0.2-0.8	200-800

	$\times 10^9$/l	/mm^3
Platelets	150-400	150,000 - 400,000

Vitamin B_{12}	200-800 ng/l	200-800 ρg/ml
Leucocyte Alkaline Phosphatase (LAP)	20-70/100 neutrophils	
ESR (Westergren) all ages, both sexes	$<$25mm/hr	
Prothrombin Time (PT)	14 sec	
PT Ratio (Test/control)	$<$1.2	

Activated Partial Thromboplastin
Time (PTT)   15 sec

Kaolin Cephalin Clotting Time
(KCCT)   40 sec

Arterial Blood

pCO_2	4.7-6.0 kPa	35-45 mmHg
pO_2	12-13.3 kPa	90-100 mmHg
pH	7.36-7.45	7.36-7.45

Cerebral Spinal Fluid

Glucose	3.3-5.0 mmol/l	60-90 mg/100 ml
Protein	0.15-.04 g/l	15-40 mg/100 ml

Miscellaneous

Faecal Fat	0.17 mmol/24 h	0-5 g/24 h
Xylose	23%/o of oral dose in 5 h more than half within the first 2 h	

Paper 1

1.1

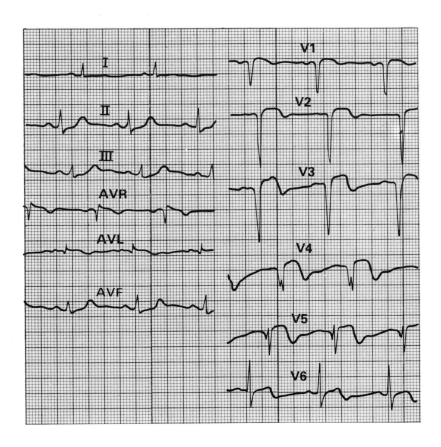

What is the diagnosis?

2

Recent Anterior Myocardial Infarction

Deep Q waves, elevated ST segments and partial T wave inversion are seen in V1 - V5. These changes are pathognomonic of recent anterior infarction. The early T wave inversion suggests the infarct is between 3 and 7 days old.

The notching of the QRS complex in V4 and V5 is due to an associated intraventricular conduction defect; **not** a bundle branch block.

1.2

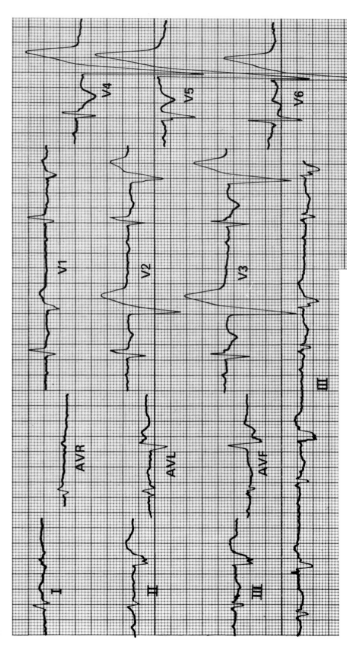

A 70-year-old man is admitted complaining of tiredness and nausea.

1. What abnormalities are present?
2. What is the cause of his symptoms?

1. a. First Degree Heart Block
The PR interval varies between 0.22 and 0.24 secs. This is prolonged.
The upper limit of normal is generally taken to be 0.22.

b. Coupled Ventricular Ectopics (bigemini)

c. Old Anterior Myocardial Infarction
In the sinus beats there is poor R wave progression in the chest leads.

d. Right Bundle Branch Block
The QRS complex is prolonged (0.12 secs) with an RSR pattern in
V1 - V4.

e. Digoxin Effect
The ST segments slope downwards leading into an inverted T wave;
the 'reversed tick' sign. This is seen in patients on cardiac glycosides
but does not necessarily indicate toxicity. The change is best shown
in the infero-lateral leads.

2. Digoxin Toxicity
Tiredness and nausea are both symptoms of digoxin toxicity. Other
symptoms that may occur include anorexia and disturbances of colour
vision of which xanthopsia is said to be the most characteristic.
Bradycardia, first degree heart block and coupled ventricular ectopics
are common features of digoxin toxicity though almost any arrhythmia
may be seen.

1.3

A 60 year old man is admitted unconscious.
Blood glucose 72 mmol/1
Sodium 154 mmol/1
Potassium 4.9 mmol/1
Bicarbonate 22 mmol/l
Total Protein 82 g/1
Osmolality 405 mmol/kg (NR: 285-295)

1. What is the diagnosis?
2. What three therapeutic measures would you institute?

1. **Hyperosmolar hyperglycaemic non-ketotic coma**
   There is gross hyperglycaemia, and dehydration shown by a high
   total protein. The low normal bicarbonate is evidence against
   ketoacidosis. The hyperosmolality is due to hyperglycaemia and
   is exacerbated by the resultant osmotic diuresis.
   Plasma osmolality may be calculated as follows:
   $(2 \times Na^+) + (2 \times K^+)$ + blood glucose + blood urea $\simeq$ plasma osmolality.

2. a. **i.v. ½ normal saline**
   Under CVP monitoring to correct the fluid deficit. Normal saline
   can be used if the sodium is less than 145 mmol/1.
   b. **i.v. Insulin Infusion** $2 - 6$ U/Hour or 5U hourly i.m.
   c. **i.v. or s.c. Heparin** in the absence of any contraindication because
   there is a high incidence of thrombotic complications in these patients.
   After the above have been instituted rigorous monitoring of blood
   sugar and electrolytes is necessary and the cause of the coma must be
   sought.

   Types of Coma in Diabetes:
   Diabetic ketoacidosis
   Non-ketotic hyperglycaemic coma
   Lactic acidosis (biguanide therapy)
   Hypoglycaemia
   Uraemic coma

1.4

A woman who had a mastectomy 10 years ago complains of backache, bruising and tiredness: She has received no treatment:
Haemoglobin 10.7g/dl
Platelets 50 x 10^9/1 (50 000/mm^3)
Prothrombin time 26 secs (control 12 secs)
Kaolin cephalin clotting time 55 secs (control 38 secs)

1. What is the haematological diagnosis?
2. Name one test to confirm your diagnosis.

1. Disseminated Intravascular Coagulation (DIC)

Probably due to carcinomatosis. Prolongation of prothrombin time
and kaolin cephalin clotting time indicates deficiency of more than
one clotting factor. This in the presence of thrombocytopenia suggests
DIC. The formation of thrombi in small blood vessels consumes
platelets and clotting factors. The fall in haemoglobin is due to haemolysis.
The process may be initiated by:
a. Release of thromboplastic factors into the blood stream from
damaged tissues.
b. Extensive endothelial damage.

Causes of DIC
Acute:
    Obstetric accidents:
        abruptio placentae
        ammiotic fluid embolism
    Heart and lung surgery
    Haemolytic transfusion reaction
    Septicaemia-especially meningococcal
    Pulmonary Embolism
    Snake Bites
    Anaphylaxis
    Diabetic Ketoacidosis
Chronic:
    Disseminated carcinoma (particularly pancreas, stomach, breast)
    Acute leukaemia
    Intrauterine foetal death

2. Fibrin Degradation Products (FDP's)

Following fibrinolysis Fibrin Degradation Products (FDP's) circulate.
Small amounts can be detected in normal people but increased amounts
circulate in DIC.
Other helpful tests include: Fibrinogen level — reduced in DIC;
Blood film — for evidence of fragmented red cells.

1.5

A woman of 50 with nausea and anorexia:
Calcium 1.63 mmol/1
Phosphate 2.50 mmol/1
Urate 0.88 mmol/1

What is the diagnosis?

Chronic Renal Failure

The high urate and phosphate are due to glomerular failure.
Hypocalcaemia in renal failure is common and may result
in osteomalacia and/or hyperparathyroidism. Factors
contributing to the hypocalcaemia include:

1. Diet. A low protein diet is low in calcium.
2. Failure of conversion of vitamin D to its most active form 1:25
   dihydroxycholecalciferol by the kidney.
3. Hyperphosphataemia. A high serum phosphate is said to cause the
   precipitation of calcium phosphate in various tissues, lowering the
   serum calcium.
4. Hypoalbuminaemia causes a lowering of total calcium although ionised
   calcium is unchanged.

1.6

A routine blood screen on a 25-year-old Greek Cypriot:
Haemoglobin 13.0 g/dl
MCV 62 fl
MCHC 28 g/dl
Film: Anisocytosis
Microcytosis
Poikilocytosis
Hypochromia
Target cells

1. What is the diagnosis?
2. What test would confirm this?

1. β Thalassaemia Minor

There are three clues here:

a. The race. β Thalassaemia minor is commonest in Mediterranean races, particularly the Greeks, where the incidence is approximately 5 per cent.

b. The film appearances. These are similar to those of iron deficiency, since both disorders are due to a failure of haem synthesis.

c. The very low MCV. The differential diagnosis in Thalassaemia minor is iron deficiency. In Thalassaemia minor there is usually only a mild anaemia in conjunction with a very low MCV, whereas in iron deficiency both fall in proportion.

The other common forms of Thalassaemia are:

(i) β Thalassaemia Major. There is a complete failure to synthesise β chains and the patient relies on HbF and HbA₂ for haemoglobinisation Presentation, even in its mildest form, occurs before the age of three with a moderately severe anaemia (Hb. 6—10g/dl) jaundice, splenome retarded growth and malleolar ulcers. Characteristic facies and X-ray changes ('hair on end') are caused by widened marrow spaces. Gallsto and haemosiderosis are relatively late complications.

(ii) α Thalassaemia Major. This is incompatible with life, α chains being necessary for the formation of foetal haemoglobin. It presents as hyd foetalis.

(iii) α Thalassaemia Minor. The haemoglobin concentration is normal and the MCV only slightly reduced. The disease is asymptomatic.

2. Haemoglobin Electrophoresis

This is the most useful diagnostic test. An increased percentage of haemoglobin A₂ is present in almost all cases of Thalassaemia Minor.

1.7

A man aged 50 complains of dyspnoea:
Vital capacity 2.3 litres
FEV_1 0.7 litres
Resting Transfer Factor 4.4 (Predicted 10.0) ml min^{-1} kPa^{-1}

What is the diagnosis?

14

Emphysema
The typical pattern of a low vital capacity with a reduced FEV_1/VC ratio is present.
Destruction of alveolar septa in emphysema reduces pulmonary diffusion capacity, hence the low transfer factor.
Other causes of a low transfer factor include:
'Alveolar/capillary block' e.g. pulmonary fibrosis
Severe ventilation/perfusion mismatch
Pulmonary congestion
Reduced pulmonary diffusion area e.g. surgical excision.
Anaemia

1.8

A 65-year-old lady with proximal muscle weakness:
Haemoglobin 12.0 g/dl
MCHC 34 g/dl
MCV 98 fl
Sodium 128 mmol/1
Potassium 4.5 mmol/1
Cholesterol 8.2 mmol/1 (NR: 3.6-7.2)

1. What is the diagnosis?
2. What would muscle biopsy show?
3. Give four other investigations you would perform to elucidate the diagnosis.

1. **Hypothyroidism**
   She has four features of the disease:
   a. **Mild anaemia with a macrocytosis.** This occurs without evidence of
      B12 or folate deficiency. The exact mechanism is uncertain, but the
      MCV returns to normal with thyroxine replacement therapy.
   b. **Hyponatraemia.** There is impaired excretion of water in severe
      myxoedema, resulting in a dilutional hyponatraemia. A number of
      mechanisms have been proposed including renal tubular dysfunction
      and disordered ADH secretion.
   c. **Hypercholesterolaemia.** Hypothyroidism is a well recognised cause
      of secondary hypercholesterolaemia. Other causes include:
      obstructive jaundice, nephrotic syndrome, diabetes, pregnancy
      and acute porphyria.
   d. **Proximal Myopathy.** Proximal muscle weakness is a common feature
      of both hyper and hypothyroidism.

2. **Type II (Fast) Fibre Atrophy**
   Type II Atrophy is a common finding in myopathies associated with
   metabolic diseases.

3. a. **Serum Thyroxine** – this will be low.
   b. **T3 Resin Uptake** – labelled T3, is added to the patient's serum and
      binds with thyroxine binding globulin (TBG) depending on the number
      of available binding sites. In hypothyroidism, as a large number of
      binding sites are available, large amounts of T3 are bound. A resin is
      then added which binds the remaining T3. If the resin count is
      measured it will be low and if, as in some laboratories, the supernatant
      count is measured it will be high.
      This test will exclude a low T4 due to deficiency of TBG e.g. due to
      nephrotic syndrome or liver disease.
      The Free Thyroxine Index can be calculated from the product of the
      thyroxine level and the resin count.
   c. **Serum TSH** – this will be high in primary hypothyroidism and low in
      hypothyroidism secondary to pituitary failure.
   d. **Thyroid Antibodies** – in view of a probable auto-immune aetiology,
      these are likely to be present in this patient. They include
      Thyroglobulin antibodies and thyroid microsomal antibodies.

1.9

A 2-month-old baby presents with fits:
Random glucose 6.4 mmol/l
Serum calcium 1.25 mmol/l
Serum phosphate 3.6 mmol/l
Alkaline Phosphatase 120 U/l
Urea 6.2 mmol/l

What is the most likely explanation?

Feeds with Undiluted Cow's Milk

There is hypocalcaemia, and hyperphosphataemia with a normal blood sugar. The alkaline phosphatase is normal for a baby. The causes of hypocalcaemia in infancy are:

1. Hypoparathyroidism
2. Secondary to hyperphosphataemia:
   High phosphate feeds, e.g. cow's milk
   Renal failure
3. Calcium or vitamin D deficiency.

Hypoparathyroidism is often accompanied by a slightly elevated serum phosphate but not of the order found in this case. This degree of hyperphosphataemia is only seen in high phosphate feeds or chronic renal failure. Significant renal failure is unlikely to be the cause as the urea is normal. Calcium or vitamin D deficiency would be associated with a normal or low rather than a high serum phosphate. In this case, as the phosphate is high, calcium phosphate is precipitated and the ionised calcium concentration reduced.

1.10

A 20-year-old girl with secondary amenorrhoea presents to Rheumatology
out-patients with painful wrists. She has slight jaundice and hepatosplenomegaly
She is on no therapy:

Hb. 13.2 g/dl
ESR 32 mm/hr
ALT (SGPT) 225 U/l (NR: < 20)
AST (SGOT) 182 U/l (NR: < 25)
Bilirubin 40 μmol/l
Alkaline phosphatase 80 U/l (NR: 20 - 100)
Anti-Nuclear Factor (ANF) positive 1/128
DNA Binding 12 U (NR: < 25)
Smooth muscle antibodies positive
LE cells negative

What is the diagnosis?

Chronic Active Hepatitis (CAH)

The clinical features and antibody screen are typical of this disease. The liver function tests show a hepatocellular jaundice. The incidence of positive antibodies in CAH is:

ANF 25-75 per cent

Raised DNA binding 5 – 20 per cent (the exact incidence has not been determined)

Smooth muscle antibodies 50 - 80 per cent

LE cells 15 per cent

The causes of hepatocellular jaundice are:

1. Infectious – e.g. 'infectious hepatitis' types A or B., infectious mononucleosis, cytomegalovirus, toxoplasmosis.
2. Toxic, e.g. alcohol, paracetamol, MAOI's.
3. Drug allergies e.g. Methyldopa, Oxyphenisatin.
4. Genetic, e.g. Wilson's disease, galactosaemia.
5. Connective tissue disease, e.g. SLE, scleroderma, ulcerative colitis.

Infectious, toxic and genetic causes give positive auto-antibodies less frequently. Hepatitis in SLE is rare and is likely to be associated with positive LE cells and a raised DNA binding.

Primary Biliary Cirrhosis (PBC) may be associated with positive smooth muscle antibodies (30 per cent) though anti-mitochondrial antibodies are more usual (90 per cent). In addition the patient with PBC usually falls into an older age group and the jaundice is cholestatic rather than hepato-cellular.

Paper 2

2.1

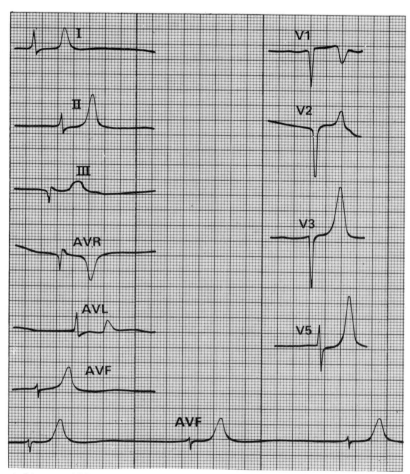

A 54-year-old becomes drowsy and confused. This is her ECG.

1. What abnormalities are present?
2. What is the diagnosis?
3. What would be your first therapeutic measure?

1. The following abnormalities are present:
   a. Profound bradycardia rate 30/min.
   b. Absent P waves.
   c. Q waves in V1 and V2 suggesting old anterior infarction.
   d. Tall, tented T waves.
      The prolonged QT interval (0.46 sec) is consistent with this degree of bradycardia.

2. **Hyperkalaemia**
   All the features listed above with the exception of (c) are typical ECG findings. The potassium was 8.4 mmol/l.

3. **Intravenous Calcium**
   10 mls of 10 per cent calcium gluconate or calcium chloride given by slow intravenous injection will reverse the ECG abnormalities and help prevent asystole.
   Other measures useful in hyperkalaemia:
   a. i.v. Dextrose and Insulin
   b. Rectal resonium — the rectal route is far more effective than the oral route as the rectal mucosa contains more exchangeable potassium.
   c. Dialysis
   d. i.v. Bicarbonate may be used with extreme care.

2.2

3

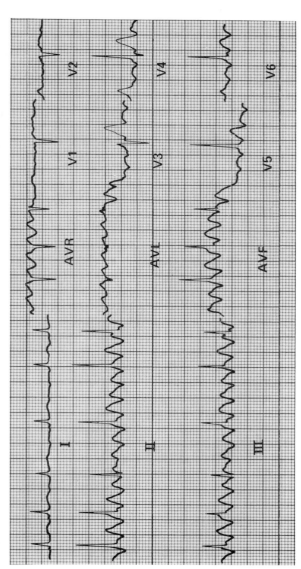

Routine ECG on a 66-year old man with an irregular pulse.

1. What abnormality is present?
2. Give the three most likely causes.

1. **Atrial Flutter with Variable Block**
   Atrial rate 300, mean ventricular rate approximately 100. Atrial activity is represented by the characteristic 'saw tooth' (wide, large voltage) waves, sometimes called flutter waves. In this case they are best seen in leads II, III and AVF. They are completely regular. The QRS complexes are irregularly spaced indicating variable degrees of conduction through the AV node. The QRS complex shows a varying conduction pattern and this is best seen in lead III.

2. **Ischaemic Heart Disease**
   Particularly following myocardial infarction.
   Digoxin Therapy
   Mitral Valve Disease
   Other causes include:
   Hypertensive Heart Disease
   Atrial Septal Defect
   Sick Sinus Syndrome
   Alcoholic Cardiomyopathy
   Other general causes of tachycardia (e.g. fever, thyrotoxicosis, tricylic antidepressant overdose) may be associated with atrial flutter in predisposed individuals.

2.3

A 42-year-old woman gives a three year history of recurrent renal colic.
She complains of 'gritty' eyes:
Calcium 3.2 mmol/l
Phosphate 0.6 mmol/l
Alkaline Phosphatase 111 U/l (NR: 20-100)
Albumin 41 g/l
Urea 8.2 mmol/l
After hydrocortisone 40 mg. t.d.s. for 10 days:
Calcium 2.95 mmol/l
Albumin 38 g/l

What is the diagnosis?

Primary Hyperparathyroidism

There are the following features:

1. Hypercalcaemia which fails to suppress (i.e. fall to below the upper limit of normal) with hydrocortisone. This occurs in:

   Primary and tertiary hyperparathyroidism

   Severe thyrotoxicosis

   Some cases of malignant disease.

   The slight fall in the calcium after hydrocortisone is in part due to fluid retention, which is reflected in the lowered serum albumin.

2. Hypophosphataemia. Hypercalcaemia with hypophosphataemia is only seen in primary and tertiary hyperparathroidism and ectopic parathormone secretion.

3. A raised alkaline phosphatase which suggests established bone disease. The length of the history (three years) suggests that primary hyperparathyroidism is the most likely diagnosis. The 'gritty' eyes are due to corneal calcification.

2.4

Following an upper respiratory infection a medical student is noticed to be icteric:

Total bilirubin 52 μmol/l
Unconjugated bilirubin 37 mol/l
ALT (SGPT) 15 U/l (NR:<20 U/l)
AST (SGOT) 21 U/l (NR:<25 U/l)
Alkaline Phosphatase 42 U/l (NR: 20-100)
Urine: bilirubin - negative
       urobilinogen - positive
Haemoglobin 15.2 g/dl
Reticulocytes 0.7 per cent

1. What is the diagnosis?
2. What treatment is available for the icterus?

1. **Gilbert's Disease**

   There is an unconjugated hyperbilirubinaemia with no evidence of haemolysis, hepatic damage or obstruction. This is a harmless congenital abnormality in which there is underactivity of Bilirubin UDP — Glucuronyl-transferase. There is a slightly prolonged bromsulphthalein retention as BSP follows a similar pathway to bilirubin. The jaundice is fluctuant and often only detectable during an intercurrent illness. The distinction from haemolysis is sometimes more difficult than in this case. Where doubt exists, further investigations, e.g. Coombs' Test, Haptoglobins and red cell survival studies may be necessary.

2. **Enzyme Inducing Agents** such as Phenobarbitone may be used. Their use is normally restricted to those with noticeable jaundice between attacks, in whom a cosmetic improvement is desired.

2.5

A 35-year-old man complains of weight loss and abdominal distention. Three years ago he was treated successfully for an itchy vesicular rash on his buttocks.

Haemoglobin 8.3 g/dl
MCHC 31 g/dl
MCV 96 fl
Film: macrocytosis+
      microcytosis+
      anisocytosis++
      poikilocytosis+

1. What is the diagnosis?
2. What investigations would confirm the diagnosis?
3. What was the rash?

1. Coeliac Disease

He has a mixed macrocytic and microcytic anaemia suggesting both iron and folate (possibly B12) deficiency. This is a characteristic feature of coeliac disease being due to upper intestinal malabsorption. Crohn's disease, small bowel lymphoma, Whipple's disease, giardiasis and partial gastrectomy could give a similar haematological picture but in this case the itchy rash should give a clue to the correct diagnosis. Remember that malabsorption due to pancreatic disease does not usually cause iron deficiency.

2. Jejunal Biopsy

A jejunal biopsy via a Crosby capsule or a duodenal biopsy via a duodenoscope would show flattening of the mucosal villi, and infiltration of the lamina propria with inflammatory cells. The abnormalities reverse when the patient is treated with a gluten free diet for a year. Some authorities claim that it is necessary to do a third biopsy after a rechallenge with gluten to be absolutely certain of the diagnosis.

3. Dermatitis Herpetiformis

This itchy vesicular rash is strongly associated with coeliac disease. It is claimed that dermatitis herpetiformis may often respond to a gluten free diet alone though dapsone is the more conventional treatment. Both dermatitis herpetiformis and coeliac disease are strongly correlated with the HLA B8 antigen.

Dimorphic Blood picture
- Coeliac
Crohns
Small bowel Lymphoma
Whipple's
Giardiasis
Partial Gastrectomy.

2.6

A 71-year-old diabetic woman with a past history of myocardial infarction becomes acutely ill:
Hb. 13.2 g/dl
WBC 11 x 10^9/l (11 000/mm^3)
Urea 9 mmol/l
Sodium 141 mmol/l
Potassium 5.4 mmol/l
Chloride 88 mmol/l
Bicarbonate 7 mmol/l
Glucose 12.3 mmol/l
Urine: glucose 1 per cent
      ketones negative

1. What is the diagnosis?
2. What two investigations should be performed?

1. **Lactic Acidosis** possibly due to Phenformin. She has a profound
   metabolic acidosis reflected in the low bicarbonate and an anion gap
   of 51 mmol/l. The anion gap is calculated as follows:

$$(Na^+ + K^+) - (Cl^- + HCO_3^-) = 51$$
$$141 \quad 5.4 \quad\quad 88 \quad 7$$

   The upper limit of normal is 20 mmol/l
   An increased anion gap is due to an excess of anions other than chlorid
   or bicarbonate.
   These anions may be:
   a. Lactate — lactic acidosis. The common causes are; shock, diabetes,
      renal failure, liver failure, phenformin, alcohol and fructose.
   b. Ketoacids — diabetes and starvation.
   c. Salicylate — in overdose.
   d. Sulphates, phosphates, organic acids — these accumulate in renal
      failure.
   In this patient the absence of detectable ketones and the near normal
   urea makes lactic acidosis the most likely diagnosis. The raised white
   count, slight elevation of potassium and hyperglycaemia are secondary
   features possibly due to dehydration and stress. Lactic acidosis due to
   Phenformin is commoner in patients with significant cardiac, renal or
   hepatic disease.

2. a. **Blood Gases**
      To confirm metabolic acidosis and determine the pH.
   b. **Blood Lactate Levels**
      To confirm the diagnosis. Blood lactate levels are usually less than
      1 mmol/l but levels greater than 5 mmol/l are necessary to produce
      acidosis.

2.7

A girl brings her four-week-old infant to your clinic with an upper
respiratory tract infection. You discover the girl has syphilis. The baby's
serology is as follows:

WR positive
FTA (Flourescent Treponemal Antibody) positive, titre 1/320
FTA IgM positive, titre 1/80

1. Does the baby have syphilis?
2. Give the reason for your answer.

1. Yes

2. A positive IgM FTA in an infant indicates active disease. Only a few false positives are described in the literature. IgM does not cross the placenta and thus this antibody cannot reach the foetus by passive transfer. It must be synthesised by the infant. Although in healthy infants IgM synthesis does not begin until the age of 6 months, in congenital syphilis it begins sooner and the FTA IgM test can be positive at birth.

2.8

A clotting screen on a boy of 10 years is as follows:
Bleeding time: 3 minutes 10 seconds
Whole blood clotting time: 15 minutes, control 8 minutes.
Prothrombin time: 13 seconds, control 12 seconds.
Activated partial thromboplastin time: 80 seconds, control 12 seconds.
Platelets 235 x 10^9/1 (235 000/mm^3)

1. What is the most likely diagnosis?
2. What investigation would confirm it?

1. Haemophilia A (factor VIII Deficiency)

A normal prothrombin time indicates functionally adequate levels of factors II, V, VII and X. The prolonged partial thromboplastin time (PTT) indicates deficiency of VIII, IX, XI or XII. The PTT may also be prolonged in the presence of a circulating inhibitor of coagulation. Factor IX deficiency (Haemophilia B or Christmas disease) is similar genetically, clinically and haematologically to haemophilia A, but is rarer.

Factor XII (Hageman factor) deficiency is also very rare and is not usually associated with clinical haemorrhagic manifestations. Factor XI deficiency resembles mild haemophilia and is extremely rare. Circulating inhibitors occur in SLE, malignant lymphoma and carcinoma. They are also found in treated haemophiliacs, (anti-factor VIII antibodies). In Von Willebrands disease the whole blood clotting time is usually normal and the bleeding time prolonged.

2. Factor VIII Assay

The disease is only severe when factor VIII levels are less than 1 per cent normal.

The thromboplastin generation test may also be performed but has largely been replaced by individual factor assays.

Normal prothrombin time = Normal levels of
II V VII X .

Partial Thromboplastin = VIII IX XI XII
Prolonged in deficiency of & + inhibitors
due to SLE, lymphoma, Ca.

2.9

A man of 50 is seen in the Cardiac Department complaining of effort dyspnoea. A heart murmur is noted.

Cardiac Catheter results:

Chamber	Pressure (mmHg)
Mean Right Atrium	3
Right Ventricle	29/3
Pulmonary Artery	28/14
Mean Pulmonary Artery Wedge	18
Left Ventricle	190/20
Aorta	110/80

Give two possible diagnoses.

1. Aortic Stenosis

2. Hypertrophic Obstructive Cardiomyopathy (HOCM)

There is a gradient of 80 mm Hg across the region of the aortic valve. This could be due to stenosis of the valve or to hypertrophy of the outflow tract — HOCM. These conditions can be distinguished by measurement of subvalvar pressure, left ventricular angiography and echocardiography.

The left ventricular end diastolic pressure is raised. This may be due to left ventricular hypertrophy (thick non-compliant muscle) or to left ventricular failure.

2.10

A man of 60 with vitiligo presents with tiredness.
He is thought to be slightly jaundiced:
Haemoglobin 6.0 g/dl
MCV 112 fl
MCHC 34 g/dl
WBC 3.9 x 10^9/l (3900/mm^3)
Bilirubin 25 μmol/l
AST (SGOT) 20 U/l (NR:<25)
ALT (SGPT) 11 U/l (NR:<20)
Alkaline phosphatase 55 U/l (NR: 20-100)
SHBD 2000 U/l

1. What is the most likely diagnosis?
2. Name three further tests necessary to confirm this diagnosis.

1. Pernicious Anaemia
There are four features:
a. Vitiligo — see below
b. Macrocytic anaemia
c. Elevation of SHBD. Elevation of this order is only found in haemolysis, leukaemia and myocardial infarction.
d. Mildly raised bilirubin in the presence of normal liver function tests, suggesting low grade haemolysis.

2. a. Bone Marrow
This would reveal megaloblastic change. Megaloblasts differ from normoblasts in being larger, and in having a more open nuclear chromatin pattern.

b. Serum B12
This would be low.

c. Schilling Test
Following saturation of B12 binding sites with intramuscular B12 1000 µg, an oral dose of 1 mg labelled B12 is given and the percentage excreted in the urine is measured over 24 hours. This will be low if absorption is impaired or in renal failure. Malabsorption of B12 due to pernicious anaemia can be corrected by concurrent administration of intrinsic factor. This forms the second part of the test.

Autoimmune Associations of Vitiligo:
Pernicious anaemia
1° Hypothyroidism
1° Hypoparathyroidism
Diabetes Mellitus
Addisons Disease
1° Gonadal Failure
Alopecia areata

Paper 3

3.1

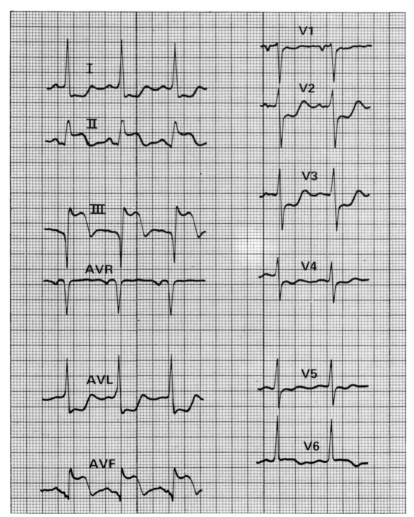

A 54-year-old woman presents with a syncopal attack associated with sweating.

1. What is the diagnosis?
2. How recent is the cardiac lesion?

42

1. **Inferior Myocardial Infarction**
   The features are:
   a. Pathological Q waves in III and AVF.
   b. ST elevation in II, III and AVF.
   c. Early T wave inversion II, III, AVF and V6.
   d. Reciprocal ST depression in I, AVL, V1 − V5.

2. **Less Than Three Days**
   The dominant abnormality is the ST elevation. If the lesion were older T wave changes would be more prominent.
   The order of appearance of ECG changes in myocardial infarction is as follows:
   a. ST elevation: 1-6 hours
   b. Q waves: approximately 24 hours.
   c. T wave changes: 2-7 days.
   The order of disappearance:
   a. ST elevation. (persistance suggests the possibility of a ventricular aneurysm)
   b. T wave inversion.
   c. Q waves. These are usually permanent.

3.2

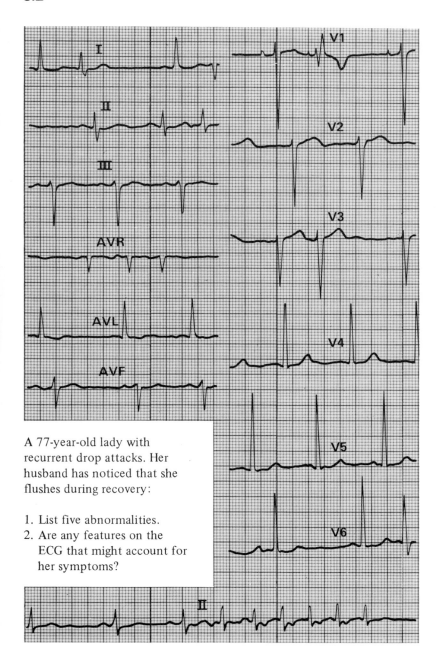

A 77-year-old lady with recurrent drop attacks. Her husband has noticed that she flushes during recovery:

1. List five abnormalities.
2. Are any features on the ECG that might account for her symptoms?

1. a. **Left Ventricular Hypertrophy**

   The height of the R wave in V5 plus the depth of the S wave in V2 exceeds 35 mm. (Sokolow's criteria). Although Sokolow's criteria of LVH are met, LVH is not present if the point system devised by Romhilt and Estes is used.

   b. **Left Axis Deviation (LAD)**

   The axis is approximately $- 30°$. The most commonly used normal range lies between 0 and +90. If the axis lies beyond -30 unequivocal LAD is present.

   c. **Atrial Ectopics**

   Some show a pattern of abberant conduction, e.g. the ectopics in V_1 which is preceded by a P wave, shows RBBB pattern and has therefore been conducted by the left bundle.

   d. **A Short Run of Atrial Tachycardia**

   Seen in lead II. The rate is approximately 170 per minute.

2. **Yes — Atrial Tachycardia.**

   The history is typical of syncope due to an arrhythmia. In this patient atrial tachycardia has been demonstrated and could be responsible for her symptoms. If there was an underlying sick sinus syndrome, other arrhythmias e.g. sinus arrest, sinus bradycardia, might be demonstrated on a 24-hour ECG tape.

3.3

A 60-year-old man has the following blood count:
Hb. 19.6 g/dl
RBC 8200 x 10^9/l (8.2 million/mm^3)
PCV 65 per cent
WBC 21 x 10^9/l (21 000/mm^3)
    Neutrophils 85 per cent
    Lymphocytes 15 per cent
Platelets 800 x 10^9/l (800 000/mm^3)
ESR 1 mm/hr
Leuocyte Alkaline Phosphatase (LAP) score 85/100 neutrophils (NR: 20-70)

He is given some treatment, recovers and is lost to follow up. He is seen
again 9 years later and his blood count is then:
Hb. 8.5 g/dl
RBC 2800 x 10^9/l (2.8 million/mm^3)
WBC 13 x 10^9/l (13 000/mm^3)
    Myeloblasts 90 per cent
    Neutrophils 2 per cent
    Polymorphs 2 per cent
    Lymphocytes 6 per cent
Platelets 45 x 10^9/l (45 000/mm^3)

1. What was the original diagnosis?
2. What was the therapy?
3. What is the current diagnosis?
4. List three other complications of the first diagnosis.

1. Polycythaemia Rubra Vera (PRV)

There is an increase in all blood cellular constituents. In secondary polycythaemia only the red cell count is raised. In PRV about 75 per cent have a raised white count and 66 per cent have a thrombocythaemi The LAP score is usually raised in PRV and normal in secondary polycythaemia, unless there is infection.

2. P^{32}

3-7 millicuries intravenously is usually sufficient to achieve remission with a fall of all indices to normal. Remissions may last from a few months to several years. In this case preliminary venesection would also have been necessary as the PCV was more than 55 per cent.

3. Acute Myeloid Leukaemia

Circulating myeloblasts in these numbers are pathognomonic of this disease. Acute leukaemia is a late complication of PRV usually occurring after about 10 years. It is possibly slightly commoner in patients who have had P^{32}, but the improved life expectancy (from about 7 years untreated to about 13 years treated) justifies its use.

4. Complications of PRV:

Thrombosis:
   myocardial infarction
   pulmonary embolism
   arterial thrombosis in any site
Haemorrhage:
   epistaxis
   post traumatic and surgical
   spontaneous — especially G.I. cutaneous and cerebral
Hypertension
Hyperuricaemia and gout
Peptic ulceration
Myelosclerosis

3.4

Thyroid function tests in a girl of 24:
Serum Thyroxine (T4) 190 nmol/l (NR: 70-160 nmol/l)
T3 Resin Uptake (T3RU) 81 per cent - supernatant not counted
(NR: 88-110)

Give two explanations.

48

Pregnancy
Oestrogen Therapy
Oral Contraceptives
These lead to an increase in Thyroxine Binding Globulin (TBG)
levels which explain the findings. Only free (unbound) thyroxine
is physiologically active. Where there is an increase in TBG
an increased amount of bound thyroxine circulates giving high
serum levels, although unbound thyroxine is normal. The most
reliable estimate of free T4 (it cannot be measured directly) may
be obtained in this case by the product of the T4 and T3RU giving
the Free Thyroxine Index (FTI). If the supernatant had been counted
the FTI would be obtained from the ratio of the two values. If the
FTI is calculated for this patient it will be seen that she is euthyroid.

Other Causes of Raised TBG:
  Congenital
  Clofibrate
  Porphyria
  Analbuminaemia

3.5

What diagnosis is suggested by the following three Paul Bunnell studies?

	No adsorption	After adsorption in ox red cells	After adsorption with guinea pig kidney
1.	+	−	+
2.	+	+	−
3.	+	−	−

+ = agglutination of sheep red cells
− = no agglutination of sheep red cells

Agglutination of sheep red cells by human serum is the result of combination of heterophile antibody with sheep red cell surface antigens.
There are three kinds which are distinguished by adsorption tests using ox red cells and guinea pig kidney.

1. Antibody that is adsorbed by ox red cells but not by guinea pig kidney is characteristic of **infectious mononucleosis.**

2. Antibody that is adsorbed by guinea pig kidney but not by ox red cells occurs in **normal individuals** and occasionally in malignant lymphoma. This is the Forssman antibody.

3. Antibody that is adsorbed by both ox red cells and guinea pig kidney occurs in **serum sickness.**

3.6

A 26-year-old man complains of night sweats and dizziness on standing.
Hb. 9.6 g/dl
MCV 84 fl
WBC 5.2 x 10^9/l (5200/mm^3)
    Polymorphs 45 per cent
    Lymphocytes 53 per cent
    Monocytes 2 per cent
ESR: 80 mm/hr
Urea 7.6 mmol/l
Sodium 129 mmol/l
Potassium 5.8 mmol/l
Blood glucose 3.2 mmol/l
MSU:
    WBC — 250 x 10^6/l
    RBC — 0 x 10^6/l
    Film — No organisms
    Culture — No growth

1. What is the underlying condition?
2. What investigations would you perform?

1. **Tuberculosis**

   He has a normocytic anaemia with a high ESR. The electrolyte abnormalities and low blood sugar are suggestive of Addison's disease. These combined with the sterile pyuria suggest tuberculosis of the adrenal glands and the renal tract.

   Chronic pyelonephritis could produce the same urinary and electrolyte findings, but would not explain the very raised ESR, and the low blood sugar.

2. a. **Synacthen Stimulation Test**

   250 mg of tetracosactrin is given. Blood is taken at 0, 30 and (in some laboratories) 60 minutes. Failure of the cortisol to rise by 200 nmol/litre (7 mg/100 ml) or to exceed 550 nmol/l (20 mg/100 ml) indicates Addison's disease.

   b. **Plain X-ray of the Abdomen**

   This may show renal or adrenal calcification.

   c. **IVP**

   To assess the extent of renal involvement.

   d. **Early Morning Urine** for microscopy and culture of acid fast bacilli.

   e. **Chest X-ray**

   f. **Sputa for Acid Fast Bacilli**

3.7

A 21 stone lady aged 30 complains of continually 'dropping off' to sleep:
Chest X-ray normal
Peak flow 350 litres/min
Haemoglobin 18.6 g/dl
WBC 6.3 x 10^9/l (6300/mm^3)
Platelets 150 x 10^9/l (150000/mm^3)

Arterial blood gases:
pO_2 8 kPa (60 mm mercury)
pCO_2 7.5 kPa (56 mm mercury)

1. What is the diagnosis?
2. Explain the raised haemoglobin.

1. **Pickwickian Syndrome**
   In this disease chronic respiratory failure is associated with gross obesity. The respiratory failure is due to hypoventilation. The cause of the hypoventilation is uncertain, but increased ventilatory effort due to obesity may be responsible. Some workers have suggested a hypothalamic lesion causing both the obesity and the hypoventilation. Primary lung disease is unlikely with a normal chest X-ray and near normal peak flow.

2. **Secondary Polycythaemia**
   This is due to the raised erythropoietin associated with prolonged hypoxaemia. Cor pulmonale is another common feature.

3.8

A 2-month-old child presents with failure to thrive, hepatomegaly
and cataracts:
Urine — positive reaction with Clinitest but negative reaction with Clinistix
Fasting blood glucose 4.4 mmol/l

1. What is the diagnosis?
2. Give two investigations which would confirm it.
3. What treatment is indicated?

1. **Galactosaemia**

   Clinitest tablets, based on Benedict's test, detect any reducing substance in the urine whereas Clinistix, containing the enzyme glucose oxidase, are specific for glucose. Reducing substances other than glucose which may occur in the urine include:
   Galactose (Galactosaemia)
   Fructose (Fructosaemia)
   Glucuronate (Drugs or their metabolites which are conjugated with glucuronic acid)
   Lactose (Lactosuria)
   Pentoses (Pentosuria)
   Homogentisic acid (Alkaptonuria)
   Cataracts are found in galactosaemia but not in the other diseases listed above. The disease is inherited as an autosomal recessive and is due to a deficiency of galactose — 1 — phosphate uridyl transferase or more rarely, galactokinase. Other clinical features include: vomiting, diarrhoea, hepatomegaly and ascites, jaundice, mental retardation, hypoglycaemia after weaning and Fanconi syndrome.

2. a. **Paper Chromatography on the urine** which may demonstrate the presence of galactose.
   b. **Measurement of Erythrocyte Galactose — 1 — Phosphate Uridyl Transferase** which will be low.

3. **Elimination of Milk and Milk Products** — the main source of galactose in the diet.

3.9

An Irish labourer presents with weight loss and diarrhoea:
Hb. 12.0 g/dl
MCV 98 fl
MCHC 35 g/dl
WBC 4.5 x 10^9/l (4500/mm^3)
Faecal fat 82 mmol/24 hr (24 grams/24 hr) on 100 gram fat diet
Xylose test 20 per cent of dose excreted in 2 hours
Fasting glucose 9.5 mmol/l
Alkaline Phosphatase 62 U/l (NR: 20-100 U/l)

1. What is the diagnosis?
2. What investigations would confirm the diagnosis?

1. Chronic Pancreatitis

There is evidence of malabsorption and mild diabetes. The malabsorption is demonstrated by steatorrhoea (normal faecal fats less than 17 mmol/24 hr 5g/24 hr). The raised MCV could be due to associated chronic alcoholism with or without folate deficiency. The main types of malabsorption are:

a. **Intestinal.** The normal xylose is against this.

b. **Biliary Obstruction.** This would be associated with a high alkaline phosphatase.

c. **Pancreatic.** The associated diabetes makes this the most likely diagnosis.

2.

a. **Plain Abdominal X-ray** — to show pancreatic calcification.

b. **Lundh Test Meal** — impaired pancreatic function may be demonstrated by reduced concentration of bicarbonate and pancreatic enzymes in the aspirate.

c. **Endoscopic Retrograde Cholangiopancreatography** (ERCP) will show tortuosity and dilatation, sometimes with stricture formation, of the main pancreatic duct and loss of the fine feathery pattern of the side ductules.

The following investigations though important in assessment are less help in diagnosis:

a. Serum folate.

b. Serum iron. This is sometimes reduced in intestinal, but not in pancreatic, malabsorption.

c. Serum calcium. } Both may be abnormal due to malabsorption

d. Prothrombin time. } of fat soluble Vitamins D and K.

e. Liver function tests. Raised liver enzymes, particularly the γ-glutamyl transpeptidase, may result from coexistent alcoholic liver disease.

f. Serum albumin.

Serum amylase is not indicated as it is normal in chronic pancreatitis except during acute exacerbations.

The fasting blood glucose is well above normal (6.6 mmol/l) and a glucose tolerance test is thus unnecessary to diagnose diabetes.

3.10

A 65-year-old lady with previously normal renal function becomes oliguric three days after a total gastrectomy for carcinoma of the stomach.

Urea 19.0 mmol/l
Sodium 130 mmol/l
Potassium 5.9 mmol/l
Urinary urea 350 mmol/l

1. What is the cause of the oliguria?
2. What treatment does she require?

1. Dehydration (Saline Depletion)

A raised plasma urea of this order in a patient with previously normal renal function is likely to be due to either dehydration or Acute Tubular Necrosis (ATN). In ATN poor glomerular filtration and impaired reabsorption of water in the tubules leads to oliguria and the formation of a dilute urine (urine/plasma urea ratio <10). In this patient the urine is concentrated with a urine/plasma ratio of 350/19 = 18.45, i.e. >10, indicating normal tubular function.
Other urinary measurements which help to distinguish pre-renal from renal failure include:

	Pre-renal	Renal
Urine Sodium (mmol/l)	<20	>40
Urine Osmolality (mmol/kg)	>500	<400
U/P Osmolality ratio	>1.5	<1.1

These tests can only be reliably interpreted in the presence of oliguria. Diuretics can increase urinary sodium and osmolality.

2. Intravenous Normal Saline.

Paper 4

4.1

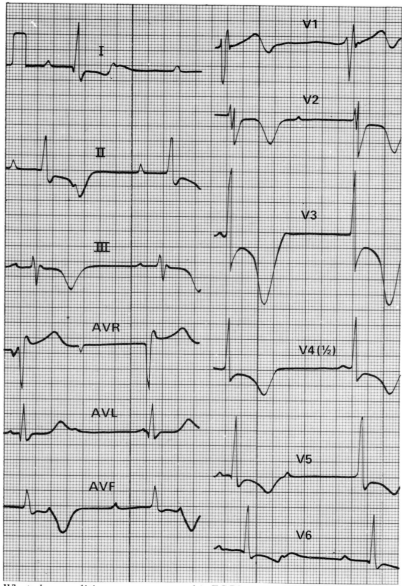

What abnormalities are present on this ECG?

1. Complete Heart Block
Atrial rate 75/min. ventricular rate 36/min. There is no fixed relationship between the P waves and QRS complexes.

2. Giant 'T' Wave Inversion
This occurs in about 5 per cent of patients with complete heart block and does not necessarily imply myocardial infarction.

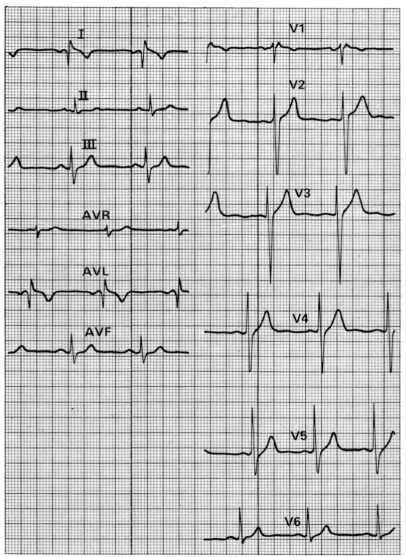

A 29-year-old man presents to Casualty with chest pain at 2 am.

How do you account for the ECG findings?

The Arm Leads have been Reversed

The clues are:

1. Isoelectric complexes in leads I and III with a positive in lead II. This combination is impossible if the leads were correctly connected.

2. An inverted PQRST in lead I. This is the mirror image of a normal tracing for this lead (right arm to left arm).

3. Apart from incomplete right bundle branch block, (a common innocent finding), the chest leads are normal.

4.3

A 35-year-old West Indian gives a 4-week history of increasing headaches and progressive blindness. Her blood pressure is found to be 210/135. She has had no treatment
Urea 35 mmol/l
Potassium 3.3 mmol/l
Sodium 130 mmol/l
Bicarbonate 10 mmol/l
Haemoglobin 9.6 g/dl

1. What is the diagnosis?
2. Why is her potassium low?

1. Malignant Hypertension

The high urea and low haemoglobin suggest chronic renal failure. The commonest causes are:

a. Chronic glomerulonephritis
b. Chronic pyelonephritis
c. Obstructive Uropathy
d. Malignant Hypertension
e. Polycystic Kidneys
f. The Collagenoses
g. Amyloid Disease

Malignant Hypertension is suggested here by the race (it is relatively common in West Indians), the history of headaches and blindness due to encephalopathy and retinopathy, and the low potassium.

2. Secondary Hyperaldosteronism

The potassium is low because of secondary hyperaldosteronism resulting in the excretion of potassium in exchange for retained sodium. Hypokalaemia can occur even in the presence of moderately severe renal failure.

Malignant hypertension causes narrowing of arterioles, particularly those supplying the juxtaglomerular apparatus. This results in low perfusion and a reflex hypersecretion of renin, which, via angiotensin causes excessive aldosterone release.

4.4

An 18-year-old secretary was found unconscious after an overdose of white tablets. She discharged herself after being given an injection in Casualty which promptly woke her up. Four days later she was admitted.
AST (SGOT) 1,200 U/l (NR <25)
ALT (SGPT) 1,800 U/l (NR <20)
Alkaline Phosphatase 180 U/l (NR 20–100)

1. What were the tablets?
2. What was the injection?

1. Distalgesic

Distalgesic contains a mixture of dextropropoxyphene and paracetamol. Dextropropoxyphene is an opiate derivative which, when taken in large doses, can cause respiratory depression, coma and cardiac arhythmias. The paracetamol component can cause a delayed hepatitis which in this case is reflected by the raised liver enzymes. The hepatitis is due to the formation of a toxic metabolite which forms a covalent bond with liver macromolecules. When present in small amounts the metabolite is removed by conguguation with flutathione (a source of SH groups) but after an overdose this mechanism is overwhelmed. Treatment with cysteamine, cysteine or methionine (all sources of SH groups) may protect the liver.

2. Naloxone

This is a potent and fast-acting narcotic antagonist, which is effective against all opiates and their derivatives. It has no intrinsic agonist activity.

4.5

A 30-year-old man develops severe left hypochondrial pain after a total hip replacement.
Pre-operative haemoglobin 12.0 g/dl
Film: 50 per cent target cells

1. What is the diagnosis?
2. Explain his hypochondrial pain.
3. Why was his hip replaced?

1. **Sickle-C Disease**
   Sickle-C disease is characterised by a mild anaemia with a very high percentage of target cells.
   Sickle cell anaemia is more severe (Hb.<9g/dl) with target forms representing 4 per cent at most of the total red cell population.
   In β-Thalassaemia Major target cells occur in larger numbers, but the disease would not have allowed the patient to survive beyond childhood. Haemoglobin-C disease occurs in Negroes and causes a mild normochromic microcytic anaemia with 30-100 per cent target cells. However, the complications described in this patients history do not occur.
   Sickle-Thalassaemia tends to produce a moderate to severe anaemia which resembles homozygous sickle cell anaemia.

2. **Splenic Infarction**
   Sickling may be precipitated by hypoxia e.g. flying in an unpressurised aircraft or anaesthesia. It may result in infarction of the spleen.

3. **Avascular Necrosis of the Femoral Head**
   Sickling may result in thrombosis in nutrient arteries. It also occurs in sickle cell disease and sickle-thalassaemia.

   Causes of target cells:
   Iron deficiency
   Liver disease
   Post-Splenectomy
   Haemoglobin-C
   Sickle-Cell anaemia
   Thalassaemia

4.6

Thyroid function tests in a man of 27:
Serum Thyroxine (T4) 50 nmol/l (NR: 70-160)
T3 Resin Uptake (T3RU) 125 per cent - supernatant not counted
  (NR: 88-110)

Give two mechanisms for these results.

1. Hypoproteinaemia (e.g. Nephrotic Syndrome)

In hypoproteinaemia there is a decrease in Thyroxine Binding Globulin (TBG) leading to a reduction in total circulating thyroxine but normal percentage saturation and free thyroxine. T3 resin uptake is increased as the total number of binding sites available to take up labelled T3 is reduced and more is available for combination with resin.

2. Concomitant Drug Therapy with Phenytoin or Salicylates

TBG concentration is normal but some of the binding sites are occupied by the drug. Fewer sites are therefore available for thyroxine so total circulating thyroxine is low and percentage saturation is reduced. However free thyroxine is normal. T3 binding to TBG is reduced as a number of the free binding sites on TBG are occupied by drug. Thus more combines with the resin, giving a high T3 resin uptake.

4.7

A woman of 55 with a rash and muscle weakness:
Sodium 142 mmol/l
Potassium 4.2 mmol/l
Calcium 2.45 mmol/l
AST (SGOT) 115 U/l (NR: <25)
Creatine phosphokinase (CPK) 750 U/l (NR: <100)

1. What is the diagnosis?
2. What diseases are associated with this disorder?

1. **Dermatomyositis**
   The patient has a rash and abnormal enzymes, probably originating from muscle. This is suggestive of dermatomyositis.
   Aldolase is another muscle enzyme that will be raised in this condition.

2. It is often associated with collagen diseases and may be a manifestation of internal malignancy, particularly in the older age group.

Causes of a Raised AST:
   Gross Elevation:
      Myocardial infarction
      Liver damage
      Muscle damage
   Mild Elevation:
      Haemolysis
      Macrocytosis
      Pulmonary embolus
      Cerebrovascular accidents

Causes of a Raised CPK:
   Myocardial infarction
   Muscle injury (including intra-muscular injection)
   Muscular dystrophies
   Myxoedema
   Severe physical exertion
   Alcoholism

4.8

Give one explanation for each of the following iron studies:
1. Fe 4 μmol/l
   TIBC 81 μmol/l

2. Fe 7 μmol/l
   TIBC 32 μmol/l

3. Fe 24 μmol/l
   TIBC 28 μmol/l

4. Fe 18 μmol/l
   TIBC 79 μmol/l

1. Iron Deficiency

A low serum iron due to iron deficiency is associated with a high TIBC (total iron binding capacity).

2. Chronic Infection, Autoimmune Disease, Malignancy and Uraemia

These conditions are often associated with a normochromic normocytic anaemia, a low serum iron and low TIBC. There is no deficiency of iron, and stainable iron stores in the bone marrow are normal.

3. Iron Overload

A high serum iron associated with a low TIBC are characteristic of iron overload. The causes are:

a. Idiopathic Haemochromatoisis.

b. Repeated Transfusions.

c. Bantu Siderosis.

A high serum iron with a low TIBC may rarely occur in liver necrosis, due to iron release from the liver stores, and in severe haemolysis where iron is released into the plasma from the R-E system following the degradation of haemoglobin.

4. Oral Contraceptive Therapy

Oral contraceptives induce an increase in TIBC. This results in an elevation of serum iron but percentage saturation remains normal. Oral contraceptives have a similar effect on thyroxine binding globulin.

low Iron high Iron binding Capacity = Iron defic.

low iron low " " " = Chronic disorders

high iron low - " " = Iron overload

high iron high " " " = Induced elevated
of iron by oestrogen

4.9

A man of 52 with a symmetrical polyarthritis complains of breathlessness;
Vital Capacity (VC) 1.8 litres
FEV_1 1.45 litres
Resting Transfer Factor 3.7 ml min-^{1} kPa-^{1}
Hb 11.2 g/dl
ESR 76 mm/hr
Rheumatoid factors: Sheep Cell Aggulination Titre (SCAT) 1/512
$\qquad$ Latex 1/2560
Anti-nuclear factor (ANF) 1/8
DNA binding 12 units (NR: < 25 units)

1. What is the underlying disease?
2. What is the cause of his breathlessness?

1. Rheumatoid Arthritis (RA)

There is a symmetrical polyarthritis with strongly positive rheumatoid factor. The presence of ANF is a common finding in RA, but the low titre of ANF and the normal DNA binding is strong evidence against systemic lupus erythematosus.

2. Pulmonary Fibrosis

There is a low vital capacity with a normal FEV1/ vital capacity ratio, i.e. a restrictive defect. This in combination with the low transfer factor, suggests pulmonary fibrosis. This is a recognised complication of RA occurring in 2 − 5 per cent of cases. It is commoner in male patients with nodules and is associated with a high titre of rheumatoid factor.

4.10

A 35-year-old man with renal colic:
Urea 8.5 mmol/l
Sodium 142 mmol/l
Potassium 2.9 mmol/l
Bicarbonate 13 mmol/l
Calcium 2.4 mmol/l
Phosphate 1.0 mmol/l
Albumin 42 g/l

What is the diagnosis?

Renal Tubular Acidosis (RTA)
There is hypokalaemic acidosis. In type 1 RTA the distal
tubule fails to acidify the urine and sodium is exchanged
for potassium instead of hydrogen ions. In type 2 RTA there
is failure of hydrogen ion excretion in the proximal tubule.
This may be associated with other features of proximal tubular
dysfunction, i.e. aminoacidaemia, renal glycosuria and
phosphaturia - Fanconi syndrome.
Acidosis leads to increased calcium ionisation with hypercalcuria
leading to nephrocalcinosis, stones and osteomalacia, though
total serum calcium is normal.
Causes of Hypokalaemic Acidosis:
a. Renal tubular acidosis
   Type 1:
      Congenital
      Chronic pyelonephritis
      Obstructive uropathy
      Hypercalcaemia
      Hypergammaglobulinaemia
      Autoimmune
   Type 2:
      Cystinosis
      Wilson's Disease
      Galactosaemia
      Fructosaemia
      Old Tetracycline
b. Acetazolamide.
c. Transplantation of ureters into the colon.
d. Partially treated diabetic coma.
e. Forced alkaline diuresis for salicylate overdose.
f. Severe diarrhoea e.g. Cholera.
NB. It should be remebered that hypokalaemia is usually associated
   with alkalosis, e.g. vomiting, diuretic therapy.

Paper 5

5.1

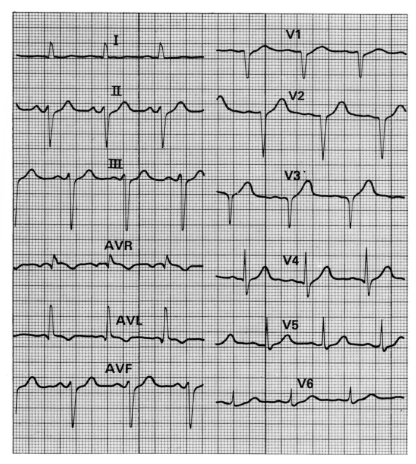

1. What abnormalities are present on the ECG?
2. What is the underlying diagnosis?

1. The following abnormalities are present:
   a. **Left Axis Deviation**
      The QRS axis is − 60 consistent with marked left axis
      deviation. This is due to left anterior hemiblock.
   b. **Q Waves in V3**
      There is definite pathological Q wave in V3 and a loss
      of R wave in V2 consistent with previous anterior
      infarction. The Q waves in AVR and AVL are not pathological
      being less than 0.2mV deep and 0.04 secs. long.
   c. **T Wave Inversion in AVL**
      The T wave axis is +90. The angle between this and
      QRS axis (the QRS-T angle) is 150°. An angle of greater than
      90° indicates significant myocardial disease.

2. **Previous anterior myocardial infarction** involving the
   anterior division of the left branch of the bundle of His
   (left anterior hemiblock).

5.2

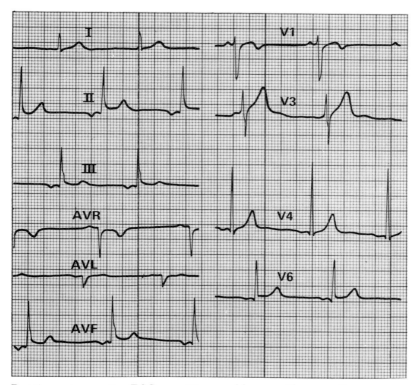

Routine pre-operative ECG on a 21-year-old man with no cardiac symptoms or signs.

1. What abnormalities (if any) are present?
2. Comment on the post-exercise ECG's.

After severe exercise: Ten minutes later:

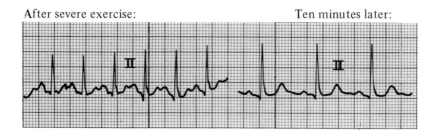

1. a. **Inverted P waves** in leads, II, III, AVF and V3 - V6.
   b. **Short PR interval** - 0.12 seconds.
   These two abnormalities suggest a resting nodal rhythm.
   Although Sokolows criteria for LVH ($SV_2 + RV_5$ >3.5 mv)
   are met, Romhilt and Estes criteria are not. (see Question 3.2).

2. **He has reverted to sinus rhythm** with normal P waves and PR
   interval of 0.16 secs.
   The resting nodal rhythm is an escape phenomenon seen in fit
   young subjects with high vagal tone causing sinus node suppression.
   Exercise causes an increase in sinus rate which then becomes the
   dominant rhythm. Atropine would have the same effect.

5.3

A 40-year-old woman with cataracts is referred from psychiatric outpatients:
Calcium 1.50 mmol/l
Phosphate 1.75 mmol/l
Urea 5.0 mmol/l

1. Give one possible diagnosis.
2. What two tests you would perform?

1. Hypoparathyroidism

A low serum calcium associated with a high phosphate in the presence of normal renal function suggests either real or functional parathormone deficiency. In hypoparathyroidism (usually autoimmune or post-surgical), there is a genuine deficiency. In pseudohypoparathyroidism there is failure of the end organs to respond normally to parathormone. Although giving an identical biochemical picture pseudohypo sents parathyroidism presents in childhood.

2. a. Serum PTH. This is low in hypoparathyroidism and high in pseudohypoparathyroidism.

b. **The Ellsworth-Howard Test** Parathormone is administered. In true hypoparathyroidism there is a marked rise in the urinary phosphate excretion and a twenty-fold increase in urinary cyclic AMP. In pseudohypoparathyroidism these changes do not occur.

5.4

A 56-year-old woman with rheumatoid arthritis has postural faints.
Blood pressure 110/60 lying, 90/50 standing. She has no oedema. Her
current treatment is indomethacin 25 mg t.d.s.
Urea 8.0 mmol/l
Sodium 130 mmol/l
Potassium 4.6 mmol/l
Urinary sodium 74 mmol/24 hours after 18 hours fluid restriction.
Synacthen test: 9 am Cortisol 731 mmol/l (NR: 170-720)
                   ½ hour after synacthen − 828 mmol/l
                   1 hour after synacthen − 800 mmol/l
Plasma aldosterone 940 pmol/l (NR: 100-330)

1. What is the underlying metabolic abnormality?
2. Name two possible causes related to her rheumatoid arthritis.

1. Salt Losing Nephritis

The patient is salt depleted. The high urinary sodium following
water deprivation (>60 mmol/24 h) points to the loss being in
the urine. This suggests a renal lesion as she is not on diuretics.
The high cortisol levels exclude Addison's disease, and with the elevated
aldosterone level, reflect the low plasma volume associated with salt
depletion.

2. a. Analgesic Nephropathy
   ### b. Amyloid Disease

Although this usually presents as the nephrotic syndrome,
salt losing nephritis may occur if the amyloid is predominantly
deposited in the tubules.

Other causes of salt losing nephritis are those where the disease
has its major effect on the tubules. They include:

Pyelonephritis
Obstructive Uropathy
Polycystic Disease
Nephrocalcinosis
Hyperuricaemia
Myeloma
Wilson's Disease
Heavy Metal Poisons
Recovery Phase of Acute Tubular Necrosis

5.5

A 23-year-old nurse complained of malaise and sore throat. Her GP gave her ampicillin which produced a rash.
Investigations at that time:
Haemoglobin 13.6 g/dl
WBC 6.2 x 10^9/1 (6200/mm^3)
Film: a few atypical lymphocytes.

Three months later she developed purpura. Repeat blood test:
Haemoglobin 12.8 g/dl
WBC 6.5 x 10^9/1 (6500/mm^3)
Platelets 15 x 10^9/1 (15000/mm^3)

1. What was her first illness?
2. What was her second illness?

1. Infectious Mononucleosis

The main manifestations in this case are:

a. Sore throat

b. Malaise

c. Rash. This is said to occur in up to 70 per cent of patients with glandular fever who are given ampicillin.

d. Atypical lymphocytes — though they may occur in other viral infections.

Other manifestations include:

Abdominal pain

Hepatitis

Splenomegaly

Pericarditis and Myocarditis

Encephalitis, Aseptic Meningitis and Peripheral Neuritis

Haemolytic Anaemia

2. Autoimmune Thrombocytopenic Purpura

This is a recognised complication of glandular fever. It is often associated with detectable anti-platelet antibodies.

5.6

A woman of 36 admitted with a DVT. On direct questioning she mentioned that her urine is occasionally dark, particularly in the morning:

Haemoglobin 11.2 g/dl
MCV 103 fl
Reticulocytes 4 per cent
WBC 3.6 x 10^9/1 (3600/mm^3)
    Neutrophils 32 per cent
    Lymphocytes 58 per cent
    Monocytes 3 per cent
    Eosinophils 7 per cent
Platelets 95 x 10^9/1 (95000/mm^3)
Leucocyte alkaline phosphatase score: 12/100 neutrophils (NR: 20-70)
Direct Coombs' test: negative
Ham's acid serum test: positive

1. What is the diagnosis?
2. Name one serious haematological complication.

1. Paroxysmal Nocturnal Haemoglobulinuria (PNH)

There is a typical history of haemoglobinuria related to sleep, and DVT is a common complication in severe cases. There is mild anaemia and reticulocytosis consistent with haemolysis. In addition there is thrombocytopenia and neutropenia with a low leucocyte alkaline phosphatase, neither of which are present in the other chronic haemoglobinurias. Typically the Coombs' test is negative. In Ham's test acidified serum is added to the patient's red cells and haemolysis occurs in patients with PNH. This is because there is an intrinsic defect in the red cells making them unduly sensitive to lysis by complement — particularly at an acid pH.

2. Marrow Aplasia

Chronic aplastic anaemia may precede, accompany or follow PNH. Occasionally an acute aplastic crisis may be precipitated by infections or blood transfusion, though a lytic crisis is rather more common. Lytic crises are also rarely caused by the administration of iron or alkalis.

5.7

Cardiac Catheter results on a woman of 45:

Chamber	Pressure (mmHg)
Right Atrium	30/15
Right Ventricle	70/15
Pulmonary Artery	70/40
End Diastolic Pulmonary Artery Wedge	35
Left Ventricle	105/5
Aorta	100/70

Give the cardiac diagnoses.

1. Mitral Stenosis

There is an end diastolic pressure gradient of 30 mm Hg across the mitral valve which is highly significant, indicating stenosis. A measurable end diastolic gradient is abnormal.

2. Pulmonary Hypertension

A pulmonary artery systolic pressure of 70 mmHg (NR: 20-30) signifies pulmonary hypertension, in this case secondary to mitral stenosis.

3. Right Ventricular Overload

The right ventricular end diastolic pressure is normally less than 5 mm Hg. The raised pressure (15 mm Hg) reflects overload resulting from pulmonary hypertension.

4. Tricuspid Regurgitation

The maximum pressure, or systolic wave, in the right atrium is very high. A pressure this high only occurs in tricuspid valve disease. As the atrial diastolic pressure is equal to the right ventricular end diastolic pressure, the lesion is probably tricuspid incompetence without stenosis. This could be functional i.e. dilatation of the valve ring, or due to intrinsic rheumatic valve disease.

5.8

A 4-month-old baby with gastro-enteritis:
Sodium 155 mmol/l.
Potassium 3.4 mmol/l
Urea 14.7 mmol/l

1. What two factors could have produced the hypernatraemia?
2. What is the first step in management of this baby?

1. a. **Intestinal Water Loss**

   In infantile gastro-enteritis the liquid stools have a low sodium content leading to predominant water deficiency resulting in haemoconcentration and hypernatraemia.

   b. **Feeding with Full Strength Artificial Feeds**

   Such foods are hypertonic. Water is lost in the stool and the solute is absorbed exacerbating the hypernatraemia. This complication is rare in breast fed babies because breast milk is less hypertonic. In contrast to conscious adults, babies are unable to say that they are thirsty. In consequence the mother may continue hypertonic fluids when water is required.

2. **Administration of Hypotonic Fluids**

   Convulsions and permanent cerebral damage can occur in hypernatraemic dehydration. The sodium level should be lowered and the water replaced by the administration of low solute fluids either orally or slowly intravenously. If the infusion is too rapid, cerebral haemorrhage may result.

5.9

A previously fit 36-year-old lady is investigated for mild hypertension and is found to have ½ per cent glycosuria. She is on no therapy.
Sodium 145 mmol/l
Potassium 3.2 mmol/l
Bicarbonate 31 mmol/l
Urea 5.6 mmol/l

1. Suggest a diagnosis.
2. Give three further investigations.

1. Cushing's Syndrome

Cushing's Syndrome is characterised by an excessive production of adrenal cortico-steroids resulting in salt retention (the mineral o-corticoid effect) and impaired glucose tolerance (the glucocorticoid effect). The mineralocorticoid effect is reflected in this case by hypertension, borderline hypernatraemia and a concomitant hypokalaemia. The glucocorticoid effect is shown by glycosuria.

The most likely underlying cause is either Cushing's Disease (pituitary dependent adrenal hyperplasia) or an adrenal adenoma.

Other possible diagnoses include:

a. Conn's syndrome. Glycosuria can occur but is very rare. The hypokalaemia tends to be more severe, with muscular weakness as a presenting symptom.

b. Ectopic ACTH secretion. The commonest causes are oat cell carcinoma of the bronchus and breast neoplasia.

2. a. Midnight and Morning Cortisols

High levels with loss of the normal diurnal rhythm is suggestive of Cushing's syndrome.

b. A two stage **dexamethasone suppression test** to establish whether the primary lesion is pituitary or adrenal.

c. **Pituitary Fossa X-ray**

Other relevant investigations include Plasma ACTH level (if available), 24 hour urine for free cortisol and total 17 − oxogenic steroids. The Metyrapone test is felt by some authorities to be hazardous and is now performed less often.

5.10

A 35-year-old housewife complains of generalised pruritus for 3 years, and pale stools for 1 year.
Bilirubin 30 μmol/l
AST (SGOT) 45 U/l (NR:< 25)
Albumin 32 g/l
Alkaline phosphatase 312 U/l (NR: 20-100)
Cholesterol 11.2 mmol/l

1. What is the diagnosis?
2. What is the cause of her pruritus?
3. Give one diagnostically useful blood test.

1. Primary Biliary Cirrhosis (PBC)
   Inflammation and fibrosis around intrahepatic bile ductules leads
   to intrahepatic cholestasis and retention of bile. This has two effects:
   a. retention of biliary constituents, particularly bilirubin
      causing jaundice, and <u>bile salts leading to pruritus</u>. It also leads
      to hypercholesterolaemia.
   b. malabsorption of fat causing steatorrhoea and deficiency of fat
      soluble vitamins.

2. Retained Bile Salts

3. Antimitochondrial antibody titre — this antibody is present in
   approximately 90 per cent of patients with PBC but not in other types
   of cholestatic or obstructive jaundice.

Paper 6

6.1

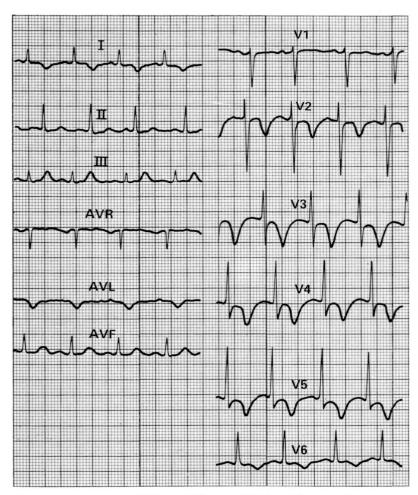

Routine pre-operative ECG on a 76-year-old lady with no cardiac symptoms or signs.

What is the diagnosis?

Antero-lateral Subendocardial Myocardial Infarction
The ECG shows sinus arrhythmia. The only significant abnormality
is the deep T wave inversion in the antero-lateral leads (I, AVL, V2-V6).
T wave inversion of this magnitude could also be caused by myocarditis
but is usually more widespread.

6.2

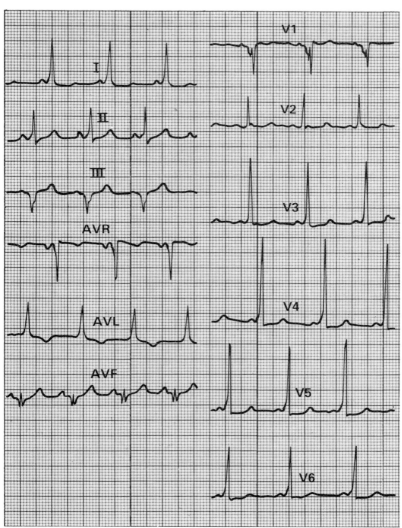

A 32-year-old woman with palpitations.

1. What are the main abnormalities?
2. What is the diagnosis?

1. There are two abnormalities:
   a. **Shortened PR interval** (0.08 s).
   b. **A delta wave is present.** This is the slurring of the upstroke of the QRS complex which is best seen in leads V5 and V6.

2. **Type B Wolfe-Parkinson-White syndrome (WPW).** In this syndrome an abnormal bundle of conduction tissue bypasses the A-V node. Impulses passing down this bundle result in the early depolarisation (preexcitation) of a part of the ventricle causing the delta wave. The rest of the QRS complex is normal as conduction via the A-V node and bundle of His occurs simultaneously.
   In Type A WPW the aberrant bundle is situated on the left giving tall R waves in V1 and V2.
   In Type B WPW the aberrant bundle is situated on the right giving a predominantly negative deflection in V1 as in this case.
   Both conditions maybe associated with frequent attacks of paroxysmal supraventricular tachycardia, the cause of her palpitations. During an attack a circus movement develops. The impulse usually travels via the A-V node and bundle of His but 're-enters' the atria via the aberrant pathway, resulting in the loss of the delta wave. This is a rhythm strip of our patient during an acute attack, which demonstrates the change.

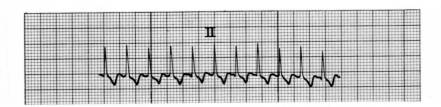

6.3

A 40-year-old man with a cough and weakness in his legs has the following CSF findings:
Pressure 11 cm H_2O
Protein 4.75 g/l
Sugar 4.0 mmol/l
Cells: RBC — none seen
WBC — a few mononuclear cells

List your differential diagnosis.

1. Guillain-Barré Syndrome

The raised CSF protein is secondary to an inflammatory exudate from nerve roots. It commonly presents with weakness in the legs, with arm and respiratory involvement occurring later (Landry's ascending paralysis). The cough could be due to an antecedent respiratory infection.

2. Froin's Syndrome

Features of this CSF are typical of Froin's syndrome with a normal pressure and grossly elevated protein content. Froin's syndrome is characterised by spinal cord compression leading to impaired venous drainage and oedema of the cord. His cough could be due to a bronchial carcinoma, with a deposit in the spinal cord.

3. Carcinomatous Neuropathy

When nerve roots are involved in this condition, the CSF protein will be high. It generally presents as a mixed sensory and motor neuropathy.

Causes of Raised CSF Protein Above 2 g/l
Guillain-Barré Syndrome
Froin's syndrome
Carcinomatous neuropathy
Neurofibromata including acoustic neuroma
Meningitis — acute bacterial
               tuberculous
               fungal

6.4

What single diagnosis could explain these findings?
Calcium 2.8 mmol/l
Phosphate 1.1 mmol/l
Alkaline Phosphatase 42 U/l (NR: 20-100)
Sodium 126 mmol/l
Potassium 5.7 mmol/l
Urea 10.0 mmol/l
Blood glucose 3.4 mmol/l

There are two possibilities:

1. **Vomiting with Dehydration**

   In vomiting hyponatraemia is due to salt and water loss with subsequent replacement with water. The hyperkalaemia and uraemia are due to poor renal perfusion secondary to hypotension. The hypoglycaemia is due to starvation and the hypercalcaemia reflects a high total protein.

2. **Addison's Disease**

   In Addison's disease, hyponatraemia and hyperkalaemia are due to failure of aldosterone induced sodium/potassium exchange in the distal convoluted tubule. The raised urea reflects the poor renal perfusion and the hypoglycaemia results from glucocorticoid deficiency. Hypercalcaemia is a recognised but ill-understood complication of Addison's disease. It is very rare but responds to treatment with steroids.

6.5

A man aged 25 with cervical lymphadenopathy complains of generalised
pruritus for 2 months:
Haemoglobin 6.0 g/dl
MCV 102 fl
MCHC 33 g/dl
WBC 8.0 x 10^9/l (8000/mm^3)
   Neutrophils 60 per cent
   Eosinophils 15 per cent
   Lymphocytes 20 per cent
   Monocytes 5 per cent
Film: Polychromasia ++
     Spherocytes +

1. What single diagnosis could explain the above?
2. Explain the anaemia.

1. Hodgkin's Disease

Lymphadenopathy, pruritus, eosinophilia and haemolytic anaemia (see below) strongly suggest a lymphoma. In a man of 25 Hodgkin's disease would be the most likely type.

2. Haemolytic Anaemia

The polychromasia and the raised MCV are due to an excess of reticulocytes in the peripheral blood. The causes of reticulocytosis are:
a. Haemolytic anaemia
b. Following acute blood loss.
   In this case, haemolysis is supported by the presence of spherocytes. Hereditary spherocytosis would explain the haematological, but not the clinical findings. Hodgkin's disease is a recognised cause of acquired autoimmune haemolytic anaemia.

Other causes of autoimmune haemolytic anaemia include:
a. Leukaemias; particularly CLL
b. Infections: e.g. Mycoplasma, infectious mononucleosis
c. Drugs: e.g. Methyldopa, penicillin, mefanamic acid
d. Connective tissue diseases: e.g. Systemic lupus erythematosus
e. Carcinomatosis.

6.6

A man of 50 presents with recurrent faints. He has an abdominal surgical scar.

Hb. 9.2 g/dl
MCV 63 fl
MCHC 24 g/dl
Glucose tolerance test:
Blood glucose 0 hours 6.0 mmol/l
½ hour 13.0 mmol/l
1 hour 10.5 mmol/l
1½ hour 2.1 mmol/l
2 hours 3.0 mmol/l

Give an explanation for these findings.

Previous Partial Gastrectomy
There is a hypochromic microcytic anaemia typical of iron deficiency.
This is a recognised late complication of partial gastrectomy, due
to intestinal hurry and failure to absorb iron.
In addition there is a lag storage GTT with late hypoglycaemia
responsible for his faints.

Complications of Gastric Surgery
Mechanical:
   early dumping
   late dumping
   afferent loop syndrome
   diarrhoea
   intestinal hurry with malabsorption
Nutritional:
   iron deficiency anaemia
   B_{12} deficiency (intrinsic factor deficiency)
   osteomalacia
   osteoporosis
Stomal ulcer
Operative complications — wound infection, pneumonia, etc.

Causes of Lag Storage GTT
Gastric surgery
Thyrotoxicosis
Severe Liver Disease
Early Diabetes Mellitus
Some normal subjects

6.7

A 44-year-old man on treatment for a 'kidney complaint' develops postural faints. His blood pressure is 110/60 lying 70/0 standing. He has pitting oedema of his ankles and sacrum.

Sodium 126 mmol/l
Potassium 4.6 mmol/l
Urea 5.0 mmol/l
Urine: protein +++

1. Is the sodium depleted or overloaded?
2. What treatment has he been receiving?
3. What treatment would be effective for his oedema and postural hyportension?

1. Sodium Overloaded

The presence of oedema means he is sodium overloaded. Postural
hypotension indicates that the intravascular space is volume depleted,
but oedema reflects an extravascular water and sodium overload
equivalent to at least 3 litres of normal saline. In this case the
maldistribution of sodium and water results from hypoproteinaemia
due to the nephrotic syndrome.

2. Diuretic Therapy

May improve the oedema but does so at the expense of the intravascular
volume and may well precipitate hypotension as in this case.

3. Protein Replacement

The underlying metabolic defect is a lowered plasma oncotic pressure
due to hypoproteinaemia. Treatment should aim to increase serum
protein levels by **(a) high protein, low salt diet.** This is minimally
effective but should always be tried as the first step in management.
(b) Intravenous Salt Poor Albumin will increase plasma oncotic
pressure with restoration of the plasma volume and a brisk diuresis.
The effect is short-lived as the albumin is rapidly lost in the urine.
It is expensive and should be reserved for patients who do not respond
to a high protein, low salt diet and diuretics.
Obviously the renal condition should be treated where possible.
However, nephrotic syndrome in adults is rarely steroid responsive.

6.8

A 19-year-old secretary is admitted in a restless and confused state.
She is pale, sweaty and tachypnoeic.
Arterial Blood gasses:
PO_2 12.6 kPa (94 mmHg)
PCO_2 3.2 kPa (24 mmHg)
pH 7.08

1. Give three possible diagnoses.
2. What immediate investigations would you perform?

1. She has a severe metabolic acidosis causing hyperventilation reflected in the low PCO_2 and raised PO_2. The causes of severe metabolic acidosis are:
   a. **Salicylate Poisoning**
   b. **Diabetic Ketoacidosis**
   c. **Renal Failure**
   d. **Lactic Acidosis** (very unusual in this age group)
   Other causes of metabolic acidosis are usually less severe. They include:
   e. Renal Tubular Acidosis
   f. Diarrhoea
   g. Acetazolamide Therapy
   h. Ureterocolic Anastomosis

2. a. **Salicylate Level**
   b. **Blood Glucose** (Test the urine)
   c. **Plasma Urea and Electrolytes**

6.9

10 years ago a woman of 50 was investigated for a goitre.
T4 232 nmol/l (NR: 70-160 nmol/l)
T3 Resin uptake (T3RU) 121 per cent (NR: 88-110)
TSH less than 0.8 mU/l (0.8-3.6)

She was lost to follow up but now presents with muscle weakness
T4 46 nmol/l
T3RU 81 per cent
TSH 22 mU/l

Give three explanations for the change in her thyroid function tests.

On presentation ten years ago she was hyperthyroid but has
subsequently developed hypothyroidism.

1. Following 1^{131} Therapy

If the patient is over 45 with a small goitre 1^{131} therapy is the
treatment of choice, but has a 40 per cent incidence of hypothyroidism
10 years later. With the advent of beta-blockers, which control
thyrotoxic symptoms, smaller doses of 1^{131} are now being used and
it is hoped that late hypothyroidism will become less frequent.

2. Following sub-total Thyroidectomy

This procedure is indicated in hyperthyroidism after failure of antithyroid drugs or when a goitre is causing pressure symptoms. It may
also be performed for cosmetic reasons. The incidence of late
hypothyroidism is between 10 − 30 per cent depending on the extent
of surgery.

3. Hashimoto's Thyroditis

This may present with thyrotoxicosis and goitre. As the disease
progresses the thyroid gland is gradually destroyed leading to
hypothyroidism.

6.10

Preliminary investigations of a 64-year-old man with a pyrexia of
unknown origin:
Hb 18.2 g/dl
RBC 7200 x 10^9/l (7.2 x 10^6/mm^3)
WBC 7.5 x 10^9/l (7500/mm^3)
   Neutrophils 65 per cent
   Lymphocytes 32 per cent
   Monocytes 3 per cent
Platelets 330 x 10^9/l (330 000/mm^3)
MSU:
   RBC $-$ 3000 x 10^6/l
   WBC $-$ 0 x 10^6/l
   No other microscopic abnormality
   Culture $-$ no growth

What is the diagnosis?

Hypernephroma
There is erythraemia (a raised red cell count) and blood in the urine.
This combination is highly suggestive of hypernephroma, with secondary
polycythaemia. Fever is a common feature of this condition. Other
causes of erythraemia are:

1. Relative polycythaemia: e.g. stress, dehydration

2. True polycythaemia:
    a. Polycythaemia Rubra Vera
    b. Secondary polycythaemia:
       Hypoxia: e.g. chronic bronchitis
       Inappropriate erythropoietin secretion: e.g. liver carcinoma,
       renal tumours or cysts, cerebellar haemangioblastoma.
    c. High affinity haemoglobin.

Paper 7

7.1

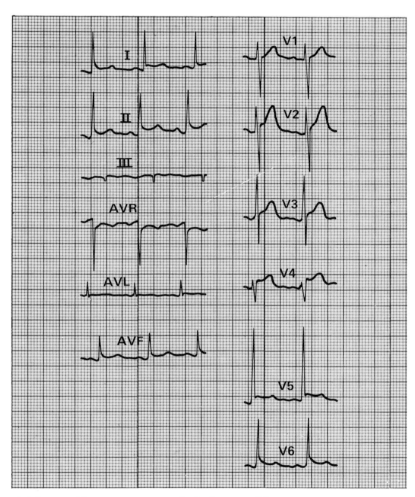

A 35-year-old man presents with tiredness and fever.

What is the diagnosis?

Pericarditis

There is widespread ST elevation concave upwards. The extensive distribution of the changes and the absence of Q waves and T wave inversion make myocardial infarction unlikely.

The causes of pericarditis include:

Infections - Viral - e.g. infectious mononucleosis, Coxackie B
              Bacterial - e.g. Staphylococal, Tuberculous
Drugs — e.g. Practolol
Inflammatory — e.g. Rheumatic Fever, SLE
              post cardiotomy and post myocardial infarction
              syndrome
Metabolic — e.g. Uraemia, hypothyroidism
Trauma
Malignancy
Radiotherapy

7.2

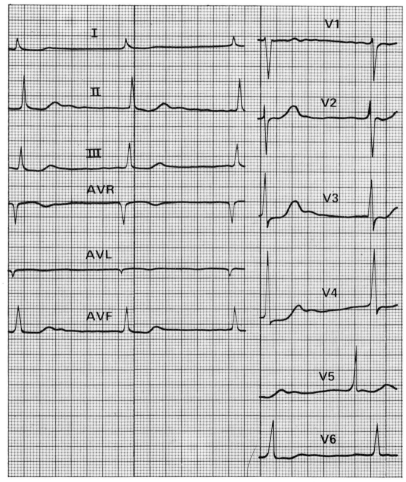

A 76-year-old man is brought into Casualty following an attack of unconsciousness. His wife has noticed a marked intellectual deterioration over the last six months.

1. Describe the main features of this ECG.
2. How would you treat this man?

1. Atrial Fibrillation with Complete Heart Block

There is a profound bradycardia rate 42/minute. The rhythm is regular but no P waves are seen. On careful examination fibrillation waves are visible in II and Vl. The atrial rhythm is therefore Atrial Fibrillation.

In the presence of atrial fibrillation a regular ventricular rhythm means that:

a. the AV node is not conducting

b. the ventricular pacemaker lies in the AV node or below.

In this case, however, the normal QRS complex indicates that the pacemaker cannot be below the division of the Bundle of His.

2. Ventricular Pacemaker

Cerebral perfusion will be improved and Stokes-Adams attacks will be prevented by pacing. A right ventricular pacemaker was inserted electively and ECG following this is shown below. It shows a pacing potential followed by a QRS complex with a left bundle block pattern.

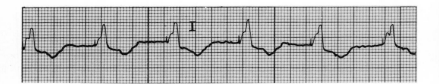

7.3

A 64-year-old man presents with hepatosplenomegaly, lymphadenopathy and retinal haemorrhages:

Hb. 11.0 g/dl
WBC 3.7 x 10^9/l (3 700/mm^3)
    Neutrophils 50 per cent
    Lymophocytes 35 per cent
    Monocytes 10 per cent
    Eosinophils 5 per cent
Platelets 105 x 10^9/l (105 000/mm^3)
ESR 110 mm/hr
Total protein 90g/l
1gG 1.2 g/l
1gA 0.8 g/l
1gM 16.8 g/l
Urine for Bence-Jones protein — positive.

1. What is the diagnosis?
2. Give a likely cause for the retinal haemorrhages.
3. Which cell type will predominate in the marrow?

1. **Waldenströms Macroglobulinaemia**
   There is a high total protein level of which a substantial proportion
   is 1gM. A rise in 1gM of this order (10 times the upper limit of normal)
   is only found in malignant paraproteinaemias. The low levels of 1gG
   and 1gA indicate an associated immune paresis. The very high ESR
   reflects the hyperglobulinaemia. The slight reduction in haemoglobin,
   white count and platelets suggest hypersplenism or marrow involvement.
   Bence-Jones proteinuria is a recognised but unusual feature of this
   disease, occurring in about 10 per cent of patients.
   High levels of monoclonal 1gM may be very rarely found in chronic
   lymphocytic leukaemia and some lymphomas.

2. **Hyperviscosity Syndrome**
   The high protein concentration may increase the blood's viscosity,
   causing slowing of the micro-circulation and sludging in the capillaries.
   This is said to be the cause of the marked haemorrhagic tendency that
   is a feature of this disease. Thrombocytopenia, impaired platelet
   function and inhibition of clotting factors may contribute to a bleeding
   tendency.

3. **Lymphocytes**
   In contrast to myeloma where plasma cells may be increased,
   Waldenströms macroglobulinaemia is characterised by an increase in
   lymphocytes in the marrow. A small proportion of these may show
   an increase in cytoplasm (plasmacytoid lymphocytes) which may be
   PAS positive, a finding of important diagnostic significance.

7.4

Investigations on a thirsty baby boy:

Plasma osmolality 310 mmol/kg (NR: 285-295 mmol/kg)
Urinary osmolality 210 mmol/kg
ADH level 18.6 ng/l (NR: 4-8 ng/l)

What is the diagnosis?

Nephrogenic Diabetes Insipidus
Dilute urine in the presence of concentrated plasma results from failure of ADH-dependent water reabsorption in the kidney, i.e. diabetes insipidus (DI). The high ADH indicates that this baby's renal tubules are unresponsive to ADH, signifying nephrogenic rather than pituitary DI. The condition is inherited as a sex-linked recessive.

Acquired nephrogenic DI may be the result of renal tubular failure from any cause, for example: Uric acid nephropathy, hypercalcaemia, Hypokalaemia, lithium.

7.5

A 24-year-old solicitor is noted to be slightly jaundiced on a routine medical examination. He has had intermittent jaundice since childhood.

Bilirubin 55 μ mol/l, 85 per cent conjugated
AST (SGOT) 17 U/l (NR: < 25)
ALT (SGPT) 12 U/l (NR: < 20)
Alkaline Phosphatase 56 U/l (NR: 20-100)

Bromsulphthalein Test (BSP):	Time	Serum Concentration
	15 min	4 mg/ml
	40 min	1.5 mg/ml
	180 min	2.3 mg/ml

1. Give a possible diagnosis.
2. How may the diagnosis be confirmed?

1. **Dubin Johnson Syndrome** (or Rotor Syndrome)
The jaundice is confirmed by a slightly raised bilirubin. Jaundice
may be prehepatic, intrahepatic or posthepatic. In prehepatic
jaundice (haemolysis) the bilirubin is mainly unconjugated. In
posthepatic jaundice the bilirubin is conjugated and there is
normally a rise in alkaline phosphatase.
In this case the lesion must be intrahepatic. Normal conjugation of
bilirubin excludes Gilbert's Disease (unconjugated hyperbilirubinaemia)
and together with normal transaminases, makes hepatitis unlikely. The
BSP test shows a normal fall in serum BSP after 40 minutes but a rise
after 180 minutes. This characteristic biphasic curve is only seen
in the Dubin Johnson and the Rotor syndromes. In these diseases there
is a failure of excretion of conjugated bilirubin (and conjugated
BSP) into the bile ductules. The second peak in the curve is thought
to be due to back-diffusion of conjugated BSP into the blood stream.
Other aspects of liver function are normal.

2. **Liver Biopsy**
In Dubin Johnson the biopsy specimen is greenish black macroscopically.
Microscopically there is centrizonal pigment deposition. In the Rotor
syndrome the liver biopsy appears normal.

7.6

Catheter blood gases in a 25-year-old man:

Chamber	Oxygen Saturation (per cent)
Right Atrium	67
Right Ventricle	65
Pulmonary Artery	70
Left Atrium	85
Left Ventricle	78
Aorta	79

1. What is the diagnosis?
2. Is surgery indicated?

**1. Ventricular Septal Defect (VSD) with a Right to Left Shunt
i.e. Eisenmengers Syndrome.**
Blood on the right side of the heart has a low PO_2 and left atrial
blood has been oxygenated in its transit through the lungs. However,
left ventricular blood is at a lower oxygen tension, indicating that
dilution with hypoxic blood has occurred. There is, therefore, a right
to left shunt at ventricular level.
   Initially in VSD the shunt is from left to right. This overloads the
pulmonary circulation leading in time to pulmonary hypertension.
Ultimately, right ventricular pressure exceeds left ventricular pressure and
the shunt reverses.

2. No
Once established a right to left shunt provides an outlet for blood
from the right heart. Closure of the defect removes this safety valve
and the pressure in the right heart rises, precipitating right ventricular
failure, which is usually fatal.

7.7

A woman of 55 complains to her GP of a 'dragging in the stomach'.
On finding massive splenomegaly he performs a blood count.
Hb. 9.6 g/dl
MCV 90 fl
Nucleated RBC 4/100
WBC 11.5 x 10^9/l (11500/mm^3)
  Neutrophils 60 per cent
  Myelocytes 6 per cent
  Metamyelocytes 2 per cent
  Myeloblasts 1 per cent
  Lymphocytes 31 per cent
Platelets 650 x 10^9/l (650 000/mm^3)

1. What is the haematological process?
2. What is the likely diagnosis?

1. **Leuco-Erythroblastic Anaemia**
   Red and white cell precursors are present in the peripheral blood
   and the haemoglobin is low.

2. **Myelofibrosis**
   Although there are a number of conditions in which splenomegaly
   and a leuco-erythroblastic anaemia are associated, Myelofibrosis is
   one condition in which both features are particularly common.
   Myelofibrosis is often asymptomatic but patients may complain of
   heaviness in the abdomen, due to the sheer bulk of the spleen. Other
   presenting features include tiredness, weight loss, pruritus, anorexia,
   gout, bone pain, jaundice and cramp.

   Causes of Leuco-Erythroblastic Anaemia
   a. **Marrow Infiltration** — due to carcinoma and chronic leukaemia
      Myelofibrosis
      Multiple Myeloma
      Malignant Lymphoma
      Lipid Storage Disease
      Marble Bone Disease
   b. **Severe Hypoxia**
   c. **Marrow Overactivity**

7.8

A woman aged 35 with exophthalmos:
Serum Thyroxine (T4) 125 nmol/l (NR: 70-160)
T3 Resin Uptake (T3RU) 101 per cent (NR: 88-110)
TRH test:

Time (mins)	Serum TSH (mU/l)
0	< 0.8
20	< 0.8
60	< 0.8

1. Give a possible diagnosis.
2. Give two further investigations.

1. There are two possible diagnoses:
   a. **T3 Toxicosis**
   Failure of the TSH to respond to TRH suggests pituitary suppression by raised levels of thyroid hormones. Since serum thyroxine is normal it is likely that tri-iodothyronine levels are raised.
   b. **Ophthalmic Graves' Disease**
   In ophthalmic Graves' disease impaired or absent TSH response may be seen in euthyroid patients.

2. a. **Serum T3** would be normal in ophthalmic Graves' disease and raised in T3 toxicosis.
   b. **1 131 Uptake** if elevated would confirm thyrotoxicosis. If the result is borderline a T3 suppression test may be performed.

7.9

A previously fit 30-year-old woman complains of tiredness:

Hb. 9.7g/dl

MCV 94 fl

Film: Microcytes
    Macrocytes
    Target cells
    Howell-Jolly bodies

WBC 4.2 x 10^9/l (4200/mm^3)
    Right shift of Neutrophils

Platelets 215 x 10^9/l (215000/mm^3)

Reticulocytes 0.8 per cent

Urea 1.9 mmol/l

Electrolytes and Liver function tests: normal

1. Explain the blood count findings
2. What is the diagnosis?

138

1. The right shift of neutrophils and macrocytosis could be due to **folate (or B$_{12}$) deficiency**. **Iron deficiency** explains the microcytes and target cells. Howell-Jolly bodies, rarely seen in megaloblastic anaemia, are a common feature of splenectomy or **splenic atrophy**. Splenic atrophy is another cause of this patients target cells.

2. **Coeliac Disease**
   The presence of a mixed deficiency anaemia and a low urea suggest malabsorption. There are also features of splenic atrophy which is a well-recognised complication of coeliac disease.

7.10

A 21-year-old man complains of haemoptysis and lassitude:
Urea 16 mmol/l
Potassium 5.1 mmol/l
Serum Albumin 21g/l
Urinary protein 5g/24 hours
Microscopy of urine: red cell casts ++

1. Give two possible diagnoses.
2. What three further investigations should be done?

1. **Goodpastures Syndrome**
   Polyarteritis Nodosa (PAN)
   (A third possibility is Wegener's granulomatosis)
   The biochemical findings of renal failure combined with heavy proteinuria and red cell casts indicate an active glomerulonephritis. The only conditions giving acute glomerulonephritis with haemoptysis in this age group are Goodpastures Syndrome, Polyarteritis Nodosa, and Wegener's granulomatosis. Bronchial carcinoma with associated glomerulonephritis (usually membranous) occurs in later life. Goodpastures syndrome has its peak incidence in the second and third decade, polyarteritis nodosa in the fifth and sixth decade. Both conditions are about three times commoner in men. Wegener's granulomatosis occurs in all age groups and is commoner in women.

2. a. **Chest X-ray** would show fluffy shadows of alveolar haemorrhages in Goodpastures Syndrome. Infiltrative shadows or pulmonary infarcts are seen in Polyarteritis and Wegener's.
   b. **Anti-Basement Membrane Antibodies** would be present in high titre in Goodpasture's and absent in Wegener's and polyarteritis.
   c. **Renal Biopsy.** In Goodpasture's syndrome there is a diffuse proliferative glomerulonephritis with linear deposits of IgG and complement visible on immunofluorescence. In PAN medium and small arteries show the characteristic segmental necrosis with a surrounding inflammatory reaction. In the glomerulus there may be focal or total necrosis. In Wegener's typical arterial wall granulomas are seen.

Paper 8

8.1

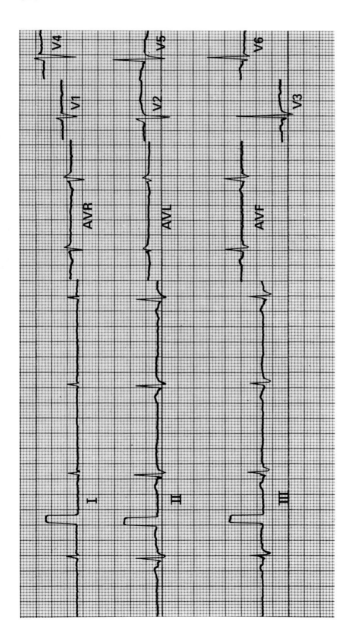

What is the diagnosis?

Hypothyroidism
The following abnormalities point to the correct diagnosis:
1. Sinus Bradycardia — rate 54/min.

2. Lowering of QRS voltage. This is usually more marked than in this ECG. It may be caused by myxoedematous changes in the myocardium, pericardial effusion, increased skin electrical resistance or by a combination of these factors.

3. Flattened T waves in all leads.
   Lengthening of the Q-T interval may also be seen in hypothyroidism but is not present on this ECG. All changes are reversed by thyroxine.

8.2

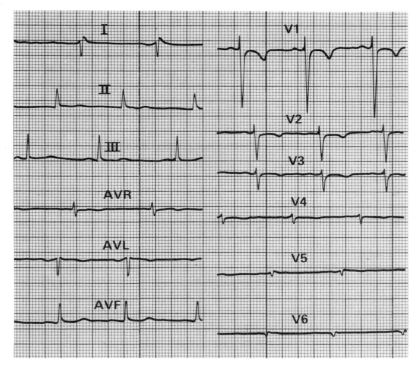

A 32-year-old man is referred to the Cardiac Clinic with an ECG taken at an insurance examination.

1. What is the diagnosis?
2. What abnormalities may be associated with this condition?

1. Dextrocardia

The following abnormalities are present:

a. Right Axis Deviation (axis greater than +90°)

The negative QRS complex in lead I with the isolectric QRS in AVR means that the axis is +120°. The causes of right axis deviation are:

   1. Right Ventricular hypertrophy e.g. mitral stenosis, cor pulmonale.

   2. Tall, asthenic subjects.

   3. Left posterior hemiblock.

   4. Secundum atrial septal defect.

   5. Dextrocardia.

b. Progressive loss of QRS voltage in the chest leads. This is only seen in dextrocardia and occurs as the exploring electrode moves further from the heart.

When right sided V leads are recorded QRS progression is normal.

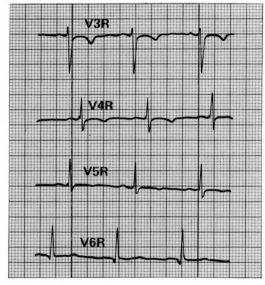

2.
a. **Situs inversus.** A complete mirror image with transposition of all viscera. Apart from their position the viscera (including the heart) are all normal.

b. **Kartagener's syndrome.** Bronchiectasis, sinusitis, dextrocardia, situs inversus.

c. **Partial Transposition of the viscera.** This is often associated with other serious cardiac abnormalities.

8.3

A 24-year-old girl complains of a painful lump in the neck following an upper respiratory tract infection. She is on no drugs:

Serum Thyroxine (T4) 175 nmol/l (NR: 70-160)

T_3 Resin Uptake (T3RU) 112 per cent (NR: 88-110)

1^{131} Uptake: 7 per cent of dose at 4 hours (NR: 11-33)

What is the diagnosis?

De Quervain's Thyroiditis

The features are:

1. A high serum thyroxine and T3RU due to high levels of circulating thyroxine. Inflammation within the thyroid gland leads to breakdown of thyroglobulin and release of thyroxine.

2. A low 1^{131} uptake due to impaired thyroid function secondary to inflammation. This contrasts with Hashimoto's thyroiditis where 1^{131} uptake parallels serum thyroxine and is thus high early in the disease.

De Quervain's is a subacute self-limiting thyroiditis. It is probably viral in origin and has been reported in association with influenza, infectious mononucleosis, measles and the common cold.

8.4

A 25 year old Asian is admitted with headache and neck stiffness.
He has been on no treatment
CSF findings:

Pressure 24 cm H_2O
RBC 0
WBC 275 x 10^6/l (275/mm^3)
Lymphocytes 80 per cent
Monocytes 10 per cent
Neutrophils 10 per cent
Protein 0.8 mmol/l
Glucose 1.8 mmol/l
WR negative

Blood glucose 5.7 mmol/l

What is the diagnosis?

Tuberculous Meningitis

There are four abnormal CSF findings:

1. CSF lymphocytosis - this occurs in:
   Tuberculous meningitis
   Viral Meningitis
   Viral encephalomyelitis (especially mumps)
   Chronic meningococcal meningitis or partially treated
     bacterial meningitis
   Cerebral abscess
   Meningovascular syphilis.
   CNS leukaemia, lymphoma
   Fungal meningitis
   Sarcoidosis

2. Lowering of CSF glucose (in the absence of hypoglycaemia). This is characteristic of bacterial meningitis but may also be rarely found in viral and fungal infections, sarcoidosis and malignancy.

3. Raised CSF protein. This can occur in any inflammatory lesion of the CNS.

4. Raised CSF pressure.

Many of the above diseases could account for the CSF findings but tuberculosis is the most likely. It is particularly common in Asians.

8.5

A 35-year-old lady with backache. X-rays show collapse of D8:
Hb 11.5 g/dl
MCV 69 gl
MCHC 24 g/dl
WBC 4.5 x 10^9/l (4 500/mm^3)
Film: right shift of neutrophils
Urea 2.4 mmol/l
Calcium 1.75 mmol/l
Phosphate 0.8 mmol/l
Alkaline Phosphatase 210 U/l (NR: 20-100)
Albumin 28 g/l

1. Why is the calcium low?
2. Explain the vertebral fracture.

1. **Malabsorption**

Apart from the low calcium there are the following features of malabsorption:

a. Hypochromic microcytic anaemia, suggesting iron deficiency.
b. A right shift of neutrophils compatible with B12 or folate deficiency.
c. Hypoalbuminaemia.
d. The low normal urea.

Other causes of hypocalcaemia include:
Hypoparathyroidism
Pseudohypoparathyroidism
Calcium and vitamin D deficiency
Chronic renal failure
Hypoalbuminaemia (including haemodilution)
Hypoparathyroidism, pseudohypoparathyroidism and chronic renal failure are characteristically associated with a raised, not low serum phosphate. In hypoalbuminaemia the calcium will fall in direct proportion to the albumin, but in this case the corrected calcium is 2.1, still significantly below the lower limit of normal.

2. **Osteomalacia Associated with Hypocalcaemia**

The low serum phosphate with the low calcium is typical of calcium and vitamin D deficiency. The raised alkaline phosphatase, due to osteoblastic overactivity, indicates the presence of osteomalacia, which is also manifested in this case by the spontaneous fracture.

8.6

A woman aged 68 complains of left loin pain. She had an abdominal operation 5 years ago:
Urea 12.5 mmol/l
Sodium 143 mmol/l
Potassium 3.1 mmol/l
Bicarbonate 15 mmol/l
Chloride 114 mmol/l

1. What operation has been performed?
2. What treatment does she require?

1. **Transplantation of Ureters into the Colon**
   The features are hypokalaemic hyperchloraemic acidosis and mild
   uraemia. The colon, unlike the bladder is capable of active transport
   of ions. Chloride is reabsorbed in exchange for bicarbonate
   producing the hyperchloraemic acidosis. Urea is split by urease-
   containing colonic coliforms releasing ammonia. This is reabsorbed and
   urea is reconstituted in the liver, creating an entero-hepatic circulation
   of urea.
   The operation is now obsolete because:
   a. metabolic complications (vide supra).
   b. ascending infection occurs frequently, giving loin pain in this patient.
   c. the technique of ileal conduit is preferred, although this may have
      the same biochemical complications.

2. a. **Potassium Bicarbonate**
   To correct the deficiencies. Requirements usually average 2-3g per
   day, and dosage is controlled by regular electrolyte estimations.
   b. **Antibiotics** — where there is clinical evidence of pyelonephritis.
   c. **Conversion to an Ileal Conduit** - where indicated e.g.,
      recurrent pyelonephritis.

8.7

A lady of 65 complains of feeling tired. She has had three attacks of
bronchitis in the last six months:
Hb. 6.7 g/dl
MCV 106 fl
Reticulocytes 25 per cent
Film: polychromasia
        spherocytosis
WBC 115 x 10^9/l (115 000/mm^3)
    neutrophils 10 per cent
    lymphocytes 90 per cent
Platelets 95 x 10^9/l (95 000/mm^3)
Direct Coombs' test: positive

1. What are the diagnoses?
2. Name two therapeutic measures you would employ.

1. a. **Autoimmune Haemolytic Anaemia**
There is a profound anaemia with a high reticulocyte count consistent with haemolysis or haemorrhage. The spherocytosis suggests haemolysis and the positive Coombs test demonstrates that the process is autoimmune. The polychromasia and macrocytosis reflect the high reticulocyte count.
   b. **Chronic Lymphatic Leukaemia (CLL)**
The very high lymphocyte count is diagnositic of CLL. Autoimmune haemolytic anaemia occurs in 10-25 per cent.

2. a. **Corticosteroids** usually rapidly control the haemolysis with a rise in haemoglobin and a falling reticulocyte count. A starting dose of 40-60 mg prednisolone a day is usual, the dose being reduced as the patient goes into remission. Corticosteroids will also lower the lymphocyte count and the thrombocytopenia of CLL may respond to steroids.
   b. **Chlorambucil** — low dose continuous treatment with this drug should aim at reducing the white blood count to around $15 \times 10^9/l$ $(15\ 000/mm^3)$

Indications for treatment:
1. Impaired marrow function: i.e. anaemia, neutropenia or thrombocytopenia.
2. Autoimmune haemolytic anaemia.
3. Marked enlargement of lymph nodes or spleen.

A high white count alone is **not** an indication for treatment.
Observation is all that is required.

8.8

A 47-year old female flower seller is admitted in late October with dark urine, pyrexia and an early diastolic murmur.
Hb 8.6 g/dl
Reticulocytes 15 per cent
WBC 15.5 x 10^9/l (15 500/mm^3)
    Neutrophils 75 per cent
    Lymphocytes 23 per cent
    Eusinophils 2 per cent
Platelets 156 x 10^9/l (156 000/mm^3)
Ham acid serum test: negative
Donath-Landsteiner test: positive
Flourescent Treponemal Antibody (FTA): positive 1/160

1. What are the diagnoses?
2. Explain the heart murmur.

1. a. Paroxysmal Cold Haemoglobinuria (PCH)

In paroxysmal cold haemoglobinuria haemolysis with haemoglobinuria is brought about by a cold haemolysin active against the patient's red cells. Acute haemolysis with anaemia, reticulocytosis, neutrophil leucocytosis, pyrexia and haemoglobinuria have been induced by the cold. In this case the time of year and occupation are obviously relevant. In the Donath-Landsteiner test clotted blood is cooled in iced water, allowing the cold haemolysin to unite with the red cells, and subsequently re-warmed when haemolysis occurs.

b. Syphilis

A positive FTA test is specific for active or inactive treponemal disease. Paroxysmal cold haemoglobinuria is said to occur in syphilis particularly in the congenital form. Other more common causes of PCH are mumps, measles and chicken pox.

2. Syphilitic Aortitis with Aortic Regurgitation

Infective endocarditis is not associated with cold haemolysins, a positive Donath-Landsteiner test or a positive FTA, though a false positive Wasserman reaction can occur.

8.9

A girl of 19 with asthma is admitted with dyspnoea. She is given 28 per cent oxygen by the casualty staff. Her dyspnoea worsens after aminophylline 250 mg i.v.
Sodium 137 mmol/l
Potassium 4.7 mmol/l
pH 7.65
Arterial blood gases:
pH 7.65
pCO_2 2.5 kPa (20 mm Hg)
pO_2 21.5 kPa (160 mmHg)
Bircarbonate 21 mmol/l

1. What is the diagnosis?
2. How would you treat this girl?

1. Hysterical Overbreathing
The classical features of respiratory alkalosis are present, namely high pH and low pCO_2. There has been insufficient time for plasma bicarbonate to drop through urinary excretion.
Causes of Respiratory Alkalosis
Hysteria
Salicylates (in association with metabolic acidosis)
Brain stem lesions
Excessive artificial ventilation

2. Reassurance
In this case overbreathing followed the correction of bronchospasm with aminophylline. Sympathetic handling was enough to relieve her apparent dyspnoea.
Alternative measures such as re-breathing or sedation should not be used except with extreme caution in an asthmatic.

8.10

A baby has had three fits, each occurring early in the morning. He is noted to have hepatomegaly:

Fasting blood glucose 2.2 mmol/l
AST (SGOT) 18 U/l (NR: <25)
Bilirubin 13 μmol/l
Alkaline Phosphatase 160 U/l (NR: 20-100)
Urate 0.78 mmol/l

1. What is the cause of the fits?
2. What is the diagnosis?
3. How is the diagnosis confirmed?
4. Comment on the alkaline phosphatase level.

1. **Hypoglycaemia**
   The tendency for the fits to occur in the early morning is related
   to the period of relative starvation which occurs overnight. The
   causes of infantile hypoglycaemia are:
   a. Idiopathic Hypoglycaemia — this probably represents a mixture
      of different metabolic abnormalities where specific enzyme deficiencies
      have not been defined.
   b. Leucine Hypersensitivity — foods containing leucine, particularly
      casein, which is found in milk products, may precipitate hypoglycaemia
      in affected individuals in the first six months of life.
   c. Glycogen storage diseases — this group consists of a number of
      diseases each characterised by a deficiency of enzymes responsible
      for glycogenolysis. Hence glycogen accumulates in the liver causing
      hepatomegaly.
   d. Hereditary Fructose intolerance — the defect causes an accumulation
      of fructose-1-phosphate which is thought to inhibit glycogenolysis and
      gluconeogenesis.
   e. Insulinomas — these occur, but are extremely rare in infancy.
   f. Babies of diabetic mothers may be hypoglycaemic in the neonatal
      period, due to foetal islet cell hyperplasia induced during intra-
      uterine life.

2. **Von Gierke's Disease** (Type I glycogen storage disease). The presence
   of hepatomegaly suggests a storage disease and the raised uric acid
   occurs only in type I. There is a deficiency of glucose-6-
   phosphatase.

3. **By demonstrating deficiency of the enzyme in a liver biopsy.**
   The glucagon test or galactose infusion test may also be used.

4. **It is normal for a growing child.**

Paper 9
9.1

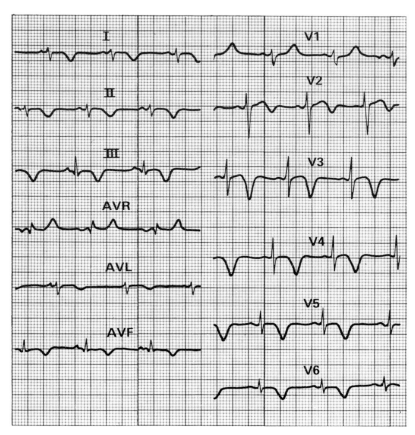

A 23-year-old girl presents with tiredness and malaise.

What is the diagnosis?

162

Myocarditis
There is widespread and deep T-wave inversion of a degree which can only occur in myocarditis or subendocardial myocardial infarction. In this case the latter is unlikely in view of the age of the patient and the extent of the T-wave changes. Although a cardiomyopathy may give this degree of T-wave inversion, this is not usual and the history suggests a viral infection. The distinction between myocarditis and a cardiomyopathy is somewhat artificial but myocarditis usually implies an infective aetiology.
The main causes are:
a. Viruses : coxsackie
influenza
infectious mononucleosis
b. Bacterial: diphtheria
rheumatic fever
c. Parasitic: Chagas disease
toxoplasmosis

9.2

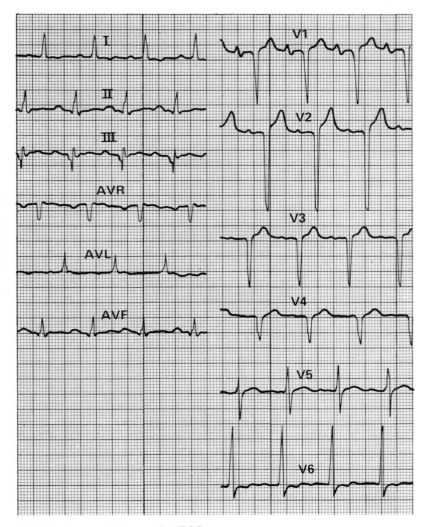

List the abnormalities on this ECG.

1. Left Atrial Hypertrophy

This is best seen in Vl where there is a biphasic P wave. The negative component of this represents prolonged left atrial depolarisation. It fulfils the criteria of left atrial hypertrophy by exceeding in 1 mm depth and 0.04 seconds in duration.

2. First Degree Heart Block

The PR interval is 0.21 seconds. The upper limit of normal is generally taken as 0.20 seconds.

3. Left Ventricular Hypertrophy

T wave inversion in the lateral chest leads (I, AVL and V6) sometimes with ST depression is a common feature of left ventricular hypertrophy. This is often referred to as 'strain' pattern.

4. Q waves in III, Vl to V4

Suggesting previous anterior and inferior infarction. The small Q wave in AVF is not strictly speaking pathological as it is less than 0.04 seconds wide and less than 2 mm deep.

9.3

A 24-year-old homosexual man is seen in a Venereology Clinic feeling unwell:
Bilirubin 35 μmol/l
Conjugated bilirubin 23 μmol/l
Alkaline Phosphatase 110 U/l (NR: 20-100)
ALT (SGPT) 750 U/l (NR: <20)
AST (SGOT) 640 U/l (NR: < 25)
WR positive

1. Give two possible diagnoses.
2. What four investigations would you perform?

166

1. a. Infective Hepatitis Type B
Type B may be sexually transmitted and is common in homosexuals as well as in drug addicts. The antigen has been isolated in semen.
b. Infectious Mononucleosis
Is spread by oral contact, is common in adolescence and frequently causes a hepatitis. A false positive WR may occur.
Rarely 2⁰ syphilis may cause a diffuse hepatitis but a miliary granulomatous form is more common. Syphilis is more common in homosexuals.

2. a. HBsAg
This will be found if the cause is type B hepatitis.
b. Fluorescent Treponemal Antibody Test
The Wasserman test may give a biological false positive in all the above conditions. The FTA test is specific for treponemal infections. Killed treponemes are used as antigen and serum is added to the slide. The antibody is then made visible by the addition of fluorescence tagged anti-human globulin.
c. Paul Bunnell
If the cause is infectious mononucleosis, heterophile antibodies agglutinating sheep red cells adsorbed by ox red cells but not by guinea pig kidney will be present.
d. Urethral Smear
Any patient with a venereal disease, should be screened for gonorrhoea and NSU.

Causes of Biological False Positive WR
Acute bacterial infection
SBE
Acute viral infection including vaccination and smallpox
Leprosy
Malaria
Malnutrition
Autoimmune diseases, e.g. SLE
Pregnancy

9.4

A man of 55 collapses outside a restaurant. He is on no drug therapy:
Sodium 115 mmol/l
Potassium 4.2 mmol/l
Urea 1.8 mmol/l
Total protein 52g/l

1. What is the underlying endocrine abnormality?
2. What test should be done to confirm your diagnosis?
3. How would you initially treat this man?

1. **Inappropriate ADH Secretion**
   There are two features of haemodilution:
   a. Low urea and total protein.
   b. Hyponatraemia.
   The causes of haemodilution are:
   a. Inappropriate ADH syndrome, which may present as epilepsy
      which in this case was the cause of the patient's collapse.
   b. Water overload.
   c. Salt depletion, e.g. loss from vomit, diarrhoea, fistulae and
      sweating, with replacement with hypotonic fluid.
   d. Renal failure.
   e. Hypothyroidism.

2. **Plasma and Urinary Osmolality**
   In inappropriate ADH secretion plasma osmolality is low and
   urinary osmolality high.

3. **Restrict water**, then treat the underlying cause.

   Causes of Inappropriate ADH Secretion
   a. Malignancy:
      Oat cell carcinoma of the bronchus
      Carcinoma of the pancreas
      Hodgkin's disease
   b. Following head injury
   c. Infections:
      Meningitis
      Pneumonia
      Pulmonary tuberculosis
   d. Drugs:
      Chlorpromazine
      Carbamazepine
   e. Acute intermittent porphyria

9.5

A man with bruising aged 50:
Urea 15.0 mmol/l
Calcium 2.8 mmol/l
Alkaline Phosphatase 84 U/l (NR: 20-100)
Total Protein 85 g/l
Albumin 30 g/l
Haemoglobin 8.0 g/dl
MCV 100 fl
Platelets 15 x 10^9/l (15 000/mm^3)
WBC 2.8 x 10^9/l (2800/mm^3).

1. What is the diagnosis?
2. Give two reasons for bruising.

1. Myeloma

The correct diagnosis is indicated by the high globulin (55 g/l) obtained by subtracting the albumin from the total protein. The other features of Myeloma in this patient are:

a. Renal failure (the raised urea)
b. Hypercalcaemia with the characteristically normal alkaline phosphatase
c. A hypoplastic anaemia which could be caused by either the disease or its treatment

2. Thrombocytopenia

Hyperviscosity Syndrome (see Question 7.3)
Low levels of plasma clotting factors would be another satisfactory explanation.

9.6

An obese male aged 56 presented with a syncopal attack associated with sweating:

Hb. 14.0 g/dl
WBC 12 x 10^9/l (12 000/mm^3)
ESR 32 mm/hr
AST (SGOT) 65 U/l (NR: <25)
ALT (SGPT) 18 U/l (NR: <20)
ECG left bundle branch block

Six weeks later his GP refers him with a PUO. His heart sounds are noted to be soft and he has a left pleural effusion.

Hb. 10.4 g/dl
ESR 108 mm/hr

1. What is the first diagnosis?
2. What is the second illness?

1. **Myocardial Infarction**
   The correct diagnosis is suggested by the raised AST (SGOT). This
   enzyme can be derived from liver, skeletal muscle, red cells or the
   myocardium. The normal ALT (SGPT) virtually excludes a hepatic
   source and the history, slight leucocytosis and moderately raised
   ESR suggest cardiac infarction. In this case the ECG is unhelpful
   as left bundle branch block may obscure anterior infarction.

2. **Post Myocardial Infarction Syndrome**
   3 weeks — 6 months following a myocardial infarction a syndrome
   consisting of fever, pericarditis (often with an effusion), anaemia
   and raised ESR may occur. This is thought to be due to development
   of anti-myocardial antibodies and results in clinical features
   indistinguishable from the well-described post-cardiotomy syndrome.
   Other features which may occur include pleurisy with effusion,
   pulmonary infiltration and ascites.

9.7

A woman of 53 suddenly starts bruising easily. She brings some pills
with her, which she has been taking for 2 years.

Hb. 8.0 g/dl

MCV 82 fl

WBC 2.1 x 10^9/l (2100/mm^3)

  Neutrophils 25 per cent

  Lymphocytes 75 per cent

Platelets 30 x 10^9/l (30000/mm^3)

Serum Thyroxine (T4) 15 nmol/l

TSH 25 mU/l

What were the pills?

There are two possibilities:
1. **Antithyroid drugs, e.g. Carbimazole, Propylthiouracil.**
2. **Phenylbutazone and related drugs.**
She has a pancytopenia which is commonly induced by
phenylbutazone and antithyroid drugs, and usually appears suddenly.
Hypothyroidism is another rare complication of phenylbutazone
therapy. Antithyroid drugs will produce hypothyroidism if used in
excessive dosage, or for prolonged periods.

Some Complications of Phenylbutazone Therapy
1. Gastrointestinal haemorrhages
2. Interference with oral anticoagulants
3. Fluid retention
4. Skin rashes, e.g. erythema multiforme
5. Nausea
6. Pancytopenia, agranulocytosis etc.
7. Hypothyroidism

9.8

A man being treated for Crohn's disease presents with tetany. He is not overbreathing.

Calcium 2.10 mmol/l
Phosphate 0.85 mmol/l
Albumin 28 g/l
Potassium 3.7 mmol/l
Bicarbonate 25 mmol/l

What is the probable cause of this man's tetany?

Hypomagnesaemia

Never forget magnesium deficiency causes symptoms very similar to hypocalcaemia. In this case the corrected calcium is normal.

Causes of Hypomagnasaemia

1. Severe prolonged diarrhoea, including fistulae, ileostomy etc.

2. Malabsorption — rarely

9.9

A 64-year-old man presents to Outpatients with lassitude. He has received no therapy.

Hb. 7.9 g/dl
MCV 84 fl
MCHC 31 g/dl
Film: Dimorphic picture of normochromic and hypochromic cells
Reticulocytes 4 per cent
WBC 4.2 x 10^9/l (4200/mm^3)
   neutrophils 65 per cent
   lymphocytes 35 per cent
Platelets 227 x 10^9/l (227000/mm^3)

1. What is the diagnosis?
2. How is the diagnosis confirmed?
3. What medication may be useful?
4. Give three possible underlying causes.

1. Sideroblastic Anaemia

He has a normochromic normocytic anaemia with a dimorphic film.
The types of dimorphism are:

a. Mixed hypochromic and normochromic, seen in sideroblastic
anaemia and partially treated iron deficiency anaemia.

b. Mixed macrocytic and microcytic which may be found in patients
with iron deficiency together with B12 of folate deficiency. Blood
transfusion may cause a dimorphic picture where there is a morpholog-
ical difference between the cells of the donor and the recipient.

2. Marrow Aspiration

The diagnosis of sideroblastic anaemia is confirmed by the finding of
ring sideroblasts in the bone marrow. These are red cell precursors with
cytoplasmic iron granules forming a ring round the nucleus.

3. Pyridoxine

Both the primary and the secondary form may respond (approximately
30 per cent)

4. Possible causes include:

Hereditary sex-linked

Acquired:

a. Primary or idiopathic

b. Secondary:

  (i) Toxic

    Alcohol

    Lead

    Antituberculous drugs

  (ii) Dyshaemopoietic

    Myeloproliferative disorders

    Haemolytic anaemia

    Megaloblastic anaemia

    Collagenoses — particularly RA

    Carcinoma

9.10

A man of 50 on no drug therapy complains of weight loss and vomiting.
Sodium 134 mmol/l
Potassium 3.0 mmol/l
Chloride 72 mmol/l
Bicarbonate 48 mmol/l
Total protein 87 g/l
Urea 12.7 mmol/l
Arterial pH 7.60

1. What is the diagnosis?
2. What is the first step in management?

1. **Pyloric Stenosis**

   Hypochloraemic alkalosis is due to loss of hydrochloric acid as a result of vomiting of pure gastric juice. When the pylorus is patent vomit contains alkaline duodenal contents in addition to gastric acid, and is of roughly normal pH.

   The hypokalaemia of pyloric stenosis is due to:
   a. Alkalosis — which causes the potassium to move intracellularly.
   b. Fluid loss in vomit leads to secondary hyperaldosteronism and increased loss of potassium in the urine.
   c. Gastric juice contains 10 mmol/l potassium.
      The high total protein and urea reflect dehydration.

2. **Correction of Fluid and Electrolyte Abnormalities by Saline and Potassium Infusion, and Naso-gastric Aspiration**

   Transfusion and parenteral feeding may be necessary later. Thereafter the appropriate surgical procedure should be considered.

   Causes of Metabolic Alkalosis
   Alkali ingestion
   Vomiting with Pyloric Stenosis
   Gastric Aspiration
   Hypokalaemia

Paper 10

10.1

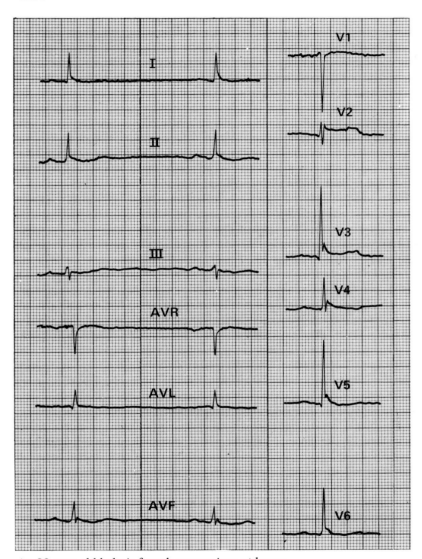

An 80-year-old lady is found unconscious at home.

1. Give five ECG abnormalities.
2. What single diagnosis could explain three of them?

1. a. **Sinus bradycardia rate 32/minute**
   b. **Muscle artefact** due to shivering
   c. **J waves.** This is a slurring of the downstroke of the QRS complex resembling a reversed J. J waves are commonly notched, as seen in V3-V5.
   d. **ST elevation** in V2 and V3.
   e. **Flattening of the T waves.**
      The long PR and QT intervals are appropriate for this degree of bradycardia.

2. **Hypothermia**
   The first three features are characteristic of hypothermia, the J wave being pathognomonic. Myxoedema, which can cause bradycardia and flattened T waves, is unlikely with normal voltage QRS complexes in the chest leads. The second ECG shows reversal of the above changes on recovery.

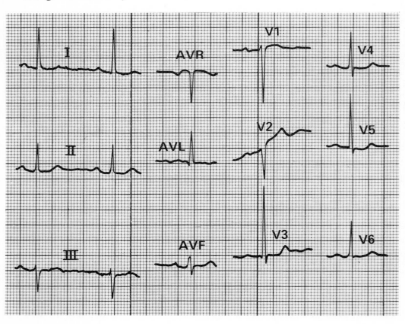

10.2

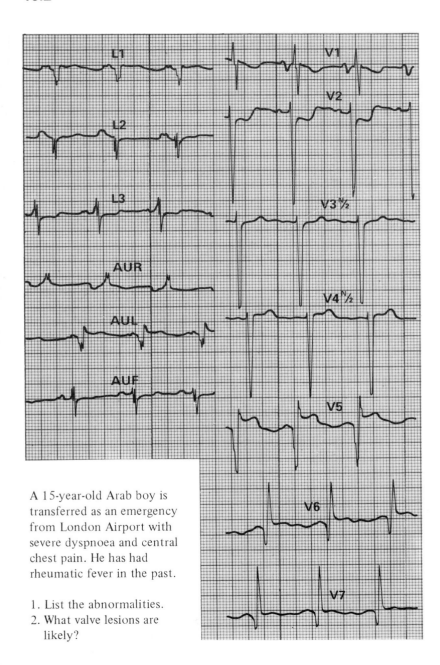

A 15-year-old Arab boy is transferred as an emergency from London Airport with severe dyspnoea and central chest pain. He has had rheumatic fever in the past.

1. List the abnormalities.
2. What valve lesions are likely?

1. a. **Left Atrial Hypertrophy**
   There is a prolonged 'M' shaped P wave in lead II and a biphasic P
   wave in V1. These meet the criteria for left atrial hypertrophy.
   (see question 9.2).
   b. **Left Ventrical Hypertrophy**
   c. **Right Ventrical Hypertrophy** is probably also present. He has
   a tall 'R' wave in V1, strain pattern in the right ventricular leads
   V1 and V2, deep S waves in leads I, II, and III and right axis deviation.
   d. **Q Waves and Raised ST Segments** in I, AVL, V5, **V6** and V7 suggesting antero-lateral infarction.
   e. **Incomplete Right Bundle Branch Block** demonstrated by RSR
   pattern in V1.

2. a. **Aortic Valve Disease**
   A myocardial infarction from any other cause would be unlikely in
   a 15-year-old boy. The diagnosis is supported by severe left ventricular
   hypertrophy.
   b. **Mitral Valve Disease**
   Although left atrial hypertrophy may occur in left ventricular
   hypertrophy or failure from any cause, changes of this degree, with
   a history of rheumatic fever, raise the possibility of associated
   mitral valve disease. Right ventricular hypertrophy provides
   additional evidence.

10.3

A 41-year-old man with headache. Skull x-ray shows an enlarged pituitary fossa:

Glucose Tolerance Test

	Blood Glucose (mmol/l)	Growth Hormone (ng/ml)
0	6.4	14.1
½ h	10.2	11.4
1 h	11.4	10.8
1½ h	10.6	12.2
2 h	9.5	12.4

Insulin Stress Test

			Cortisol (nmol/l)
0	7.2	14.1	380
½ h	2.1	15.2	410
45 m	1.8	14.8	405
1 h	2.5	15.4	407
1½ h	4.6	15.2	395

1. What endocrine abnormalities are present?
2. What other tests should be performed?

1. The following endocrine abnormalities are present:
   a. **Growth Hormone Excess** (Acromegaly)
      The resting growth hormone level is elevated (>10ng/ml) and
      fails to suppress (fall to <5ng/ml) during the glucose tolerance test.
   b. **Diabetes Mellitus**
      There is a diabetic glucose tolerance curve, with a one hour blood
      glucose greater than 9.2 mmols/l and a two-hour blood glucose greater
      than 6.6 mmol/l. The diabetes is probably secondary to acromegaly.
   c. **Cortisol Deficiency**
      The cortisol fails to rise above 570 nmol/l during the Insulin Stress
      Test, although adequate hypoglycaemia (<2.2 mmol/l) has been
      obtained. In the presence of acromegaly this is likely to result from
      pituitary rather than adrenal dysfunction.

2. The following tests should be performed:
   a. Tests to assess the size of the tumour
      EMI scan: to assess whether the tumour has a suprasellar
      extension. This test, where available, is an alternative to
      air encephalography.
   b: Tests to assess endocrine function.
      Gonadotrophin levels
      LHRH Test if gonadotrophin levels are borderline.
      Prolactin Levels
      Thyroxine and TSH levels
      Synacthen Stimulation Test To confirm that the cortisol
      deficiency is pituitary in origin.
   c. Tests useful in monitoring
      X-ray of the heel — to assess heel pad thickness.
      Hand and foot volumes.

10.4

A boy of 6 from Glasgow is admitted with abdominal pain and
constipation. There are no skin lesions.
Hb. 9.1 g/dl
MCV 86 fl
Urea 10.7 mmol/l
Urine: δ-amino-laevulinic acid present
  24-hour urinary coproporphyrin 0.17 mg (NR: <0.1)

1. What is the diagnosis?
2. List three complications that can occur.

188

1. Lead Poisoning

There is a normocytic anaemia. Punctuate basophilia due to precipitated RNA in the red cell is often present, but is not specific for lead poisoning. It also occurs in pernicious anaemia, leukaemias and many of the haemoglobinopathies. The absence of skin lesions excludes congenital erythropoetic porphyria, the only variant in which anaemia is a feature. The raised urea is evidence of the nephro-toxicity of lead. Lead inhibits the formation of δ-amino-laevulinic acid (δ-ALA), its conversion to porphobilinogen and the incorporation of iron into protoporphyrin to form haem. This leads to the accumulation of δ-ALA and coproporphyrin III in the blood and their excretion in the urine. Failure of incorporation of iron may lead to a sideroblastic anaemia. Lead poisoning is relatively common in Glasgow where exposure to lead in water (lead pipes), paint and car exhaust fumes is frequent.

2. Anaemia
Nephrotoxicity
Encephalopathy
Peripheral Neuropathy
are all complications of lead poisoning.

10.5

A woman of 45 years has a blood pressure of 200/130.
Urinary Hydroxy - Methoxy - Mandelic Acid (HMMA)
75 υmol/24 hours (NR: 5-35)

Give four possible explanations.

1. **Phaeochromocytoma**
   This causes high levels of urinary catecholamine breakdown products metanephrine, nor-metanephrine or hydroxy-methoxy-mandelic acid.

2. **Clonidine Withdrawal**
   It is now well-recognised that sudden cessation of clonidine therapy leads to a hypertensive crisis with high plasma and urinary catecholamines.

3. **Methyldopa Therapy**
   Methyldopa and its metabolites may give falsely high values by interfering with the assay.

4. **Monoamine Oxidase Inhibitors**
   The ingestion of sympathomimetic amines, e.g. tyramine containing foods, ephedrine etc, lead to the release of endogenous catecholamines giving high urinary and plasma catecholamine levels.

   Other Causes of a Raised Urinary HMMA:

Foods	Drugs
Bananas	Tetracyclines
Ice cream	Phenothiazines
Tea	
Coffee	
Chocolate	
Vanilla	

10.6

A 45-year-old lady with rheumatoid arthritis (RA) has a haemoglobin of 9.5 g/dl.

Give five possible explanations.

1. Anaemia of chronic disorders
   In RA anaemia is an important manifestation of active disease.
   It may be normocytic, or microcytic even in the absence of iron
   deficiency. A frank sideroblastic anaemia may occur in severe cases.

2. Iron Deficiency
   There is an increased incidence of peptic ulceration in RA, which
   may cause chronic gastrointestinal blood loss. Many of the commonly
   used anti-inflammatory drugs such as aspirin, phenylbutazone and
   indomethacin also cause GI bleeding.

3. Hypoplastic Anaemia
   This is a rare but important complication of phenylbutazone,
   indomethacin, gold and penicillamine.

4. Felty's Syndrome
   Anaemia, thrombocytopenia and leucopenia occur secondary to
   hypersplenism.

5. Renal Failure
   Renal failure may occur as a result of amyloid disease, analgesic
   nephropathy or rarely an immune-complex glomerulonephritis which
   may be induced by penicillamine.

10.7

A 35-year-old patient who has been on haemodialysis for 10 years complains of bone pain. He has been on no drugs except for aluminium hydroxide tablets.
Pre-dialysis results:
Calcium 3.5 mmol/l
Phosphate 0.6 mmol/l
Alkaline Phosphatase 350 U/l (NR: 20-100)

1. What is the most likely diagnosis?
2. What treatment would correct the disorder?

1. **Tertiary Hyperparathyroidism**
   The patient is hypercalcaemic with a high alkaline phosphatase and a low phosphate. The level of phosphate varies in renal failure, being influenced by:
   a. Dialysis
   b. Diet
   c. Treatment with aluminium hydroxide — which forms insoluble aluminium phosphate in the gut, thus preventing phosphate absorption
   d. Parathormone levels.
   Secondary hyperparathyroidism is common in long standing renal failure, and results from hypocalcaemia. (see question 1.5).
   In secondary hyperparathyroidism parathormone secretion remains appropriate to the level of calcium. However, after prolonged feedback stimulation, parathormone secretion may become autonomous and lead to hypercalcaemia.
   The raised alkaline phosphatase is due to the associated bone disease.
   Tertiary hyperparathyroidism is not uncommon in patients on long-term haemodialysis.

2. **Subtotal parathyroidectomy**, or removal of the parathyroid adenoma if present.

10.8

A 35-year-old woman with Crohn's disease is investigated for anaemia:
Hb. 8.0 g/dl
MCV 112 fl
Film: Macrocytosis ++
Serum B_{12} 80ng/l (NR: >200)

Schilling Test	Percentage Oral dose excreted in the urine
Part 1 (without intrinsic factor)	3.1 per cent
Part 11 (with intrinsic factor)	3.5 per cent
After 10 days of treatment with oxytetra-cycline repeat Part 1	11.4 per cent

1. What is the underlying cause of her anaemia?
2. What other investigations are useful in making this diagnosis?

1. Blind Loop Syndrome

She has a macrocytic anaemia due to Vitamin B_{12} deficiency. The causes of B_{12} deficiency are:

a. Absence of intrinsic factor.

Due to intrinsic factor or gastric parietal cell antibodies — pernicious anaemia.

Following total gastrectomy.

b. Disease of the Terminal Ileum (the area where B_{12} is absorbed) e.g. Crohn's disease, surgical resection.

c. Competition for B_{12} absorption.

Blind loop syndrome.

Fish tape worm.

In the Schilling test 1 mg of radiolabelled B_{12} is given orally with a simultaneous injection 1000 mg of cyanocobalamin. Urine is collected for 24 hours and the percentage of absorbed B_{12} is calculated by measuring the proportion of the radiolabel that appears in the urine. If the amount is 5 per cent or less there is significant malabsorption of B12.

In pernicious anaemia or following gastrectomy B_{12} malabsorption is corrected by intrinsic factor. In terminal ileal disease absorption remains impaired after either intrinsic factor or antibiotics.

In blind loop syndrome (a common feature of Crohn's disease) overgrowth of bacteria occurs in parts of the bowel where there is stagnation of intestinal contents. This may occur in diverticula or in loops of bowel which have been bypassed either surgically or following the development of fistulae. The overgrowth of bacteria (usually anaerobes) compete for the absorption of B_{12} resulting in a deficiency of the vitamin. Oral tetracycline reduces the number of organisms and B_{12} absorption is returned to normal.

2. a. Barium Meal and Follow Through

b. **Urinary Indican.** Tryptophan in broken down to indole by the bacteria. This is then absorbed, converted to indican by the liver and excreted in the urine. The amount of urinary indican reflects the degree of bacterial overgrowth in the blind loop.

c. **C^{14} Breath Test.** C^{14} labelled conjugated bile salts are given orally. In the presence of bacterial overgrowth these are deconjugated and the amino-acid reabsorbed and metabolised forming carbon dioxide. The radiolabelled carbon component of the carbon dioxide may be measured in the breath. High levels occur in blind loop syndrome and in terminal ileum disease.

d. **Direct Sampling and Culture of Intestinal Contents.**

10.9

A 65-year-old woman treated for hypertension for 20 years complains
of tiredness and shortness of breath:
Haemoglobin 8.0 g/dl
MCV 98 fl
Film: Polychromasia
    Spherocytosis

1. What is the probable diagnosis?
2. What two tests would confirm it?

1. Methyldopa-induced Haemolytic Anaemia

The polychromasia and raised MCV is due to an excess of reticulocytes. Although there are many other causes for anaemia with a reticulocytosis the history of longstanding treatment for hypertension should give the correct diagnosis.

Approximately 20 per cent of patients on methyldopa therapy for more than 1 year develop a positive Coombs' Test, but overt signs of haemolysis occur in less than 1 per cent.

2. a. Reticulocyte count
   b. Coombs' Test.

10.10

A maniac-depressive of 30 complains of thirst. She is apparently well controlled with lithium:
Serum lithium 0.85 mmol/l (therapeutic range 0.7 - 1.4 mmol/l)
After an 8 hour water deprivation test:
Urinary osmolality 300 mmol/kg
Plasma osmolality 295 mmol/kg (NR: 285-295)

After 20 g des-amino d-arginine vasopressin (DDAVP) intranasally
Urinary osmolality 335 mmol/kg
Plasma osmolality 300 mmol/kg

What is the diagnosis?

Nephrogenic Diabetes Insipidus (DI) due to Lithium
During a water deprivation test plasma osmolality should not exceed
300 mmol/l and urinary osmolality should exceed 600 mmol/l
(i.e. twice the plasma osmolality). Failure of this normal response
indicates diabetes insipidus.
In psychogenic polydipsia furtive water ingestion during a deprivation
test may lead to failure of urine concentration but plasma osmolality will
remain normal or fall.
Failure of urinary concentration following DDAVP indicates renal
insensitivity to ADH; i.e. nephrogenic diabetes insipidus. In cranial
DI the abnormalities would be corrected by DDAVP.
Nephrogenic DI may be caused by lithium even when the serum levels are
within the therapeutic range.